I0120809

LIVING AN INSPIRED LIFE

Walking in step with the Author of All Things

2026

DANIEL & VICKI HAGADORN

Living An Inspired Life: Walking in step with the Author of All Things

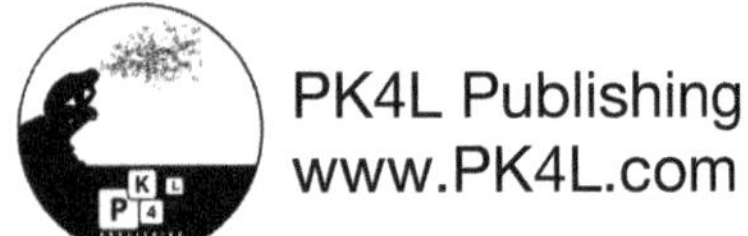

PK4L Publishing
www.PK4L.com

Inspired Life
getinspiredmovement@gmail.com

Every attempt has been made to source all quotes properly.

ISBN: 978-0-9992827-7-9

10 9 8 7 6 5 4 3 2 1

First Printing, 2021

Printed in the United States of America

CONTENTS

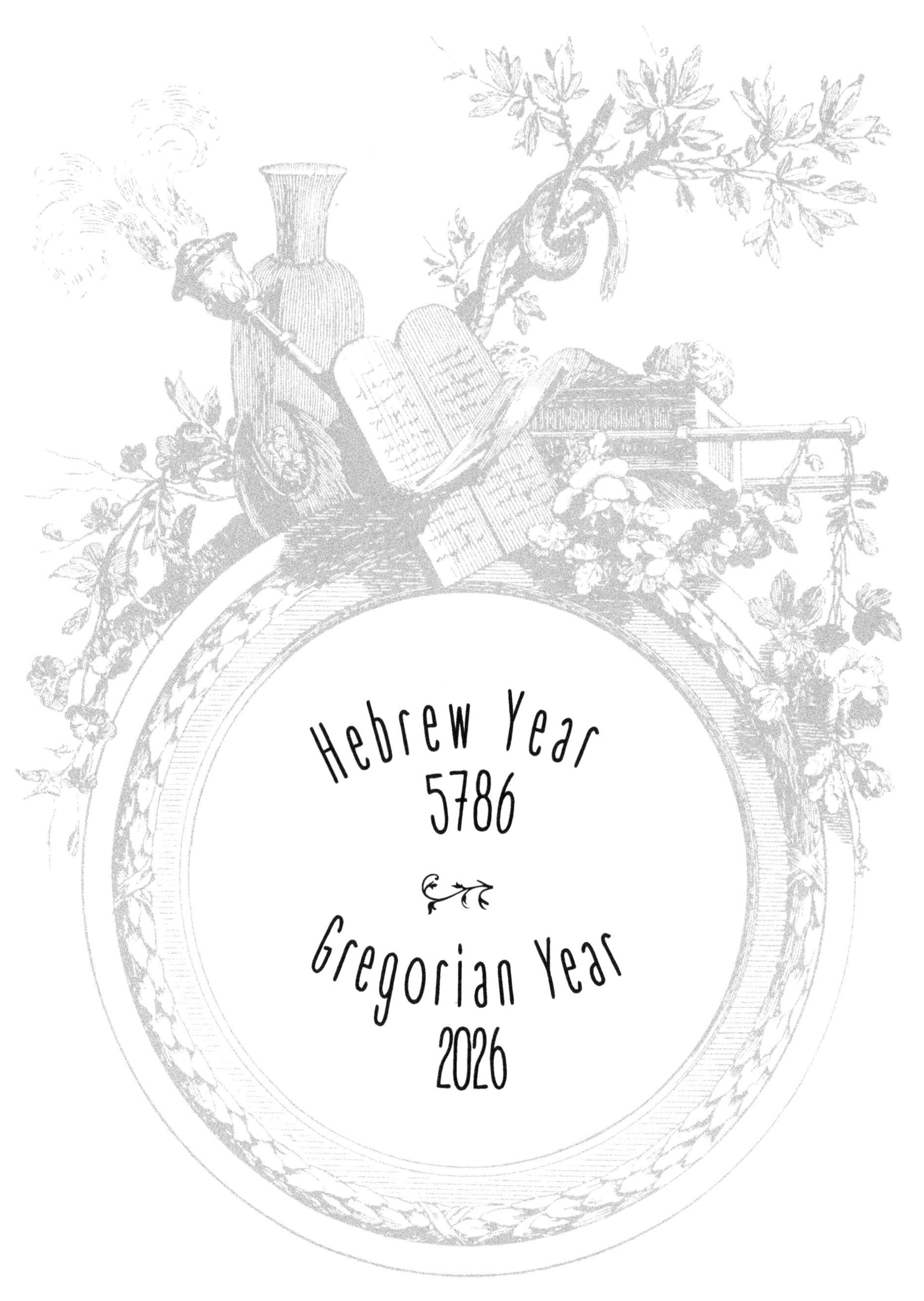
Hebrew Year
5786
Gregorian Year
2026

PROLOGUE

Welcome to the updated edition of the Inspired Life Guide! As we enter the Hebrew year 5786, we invite you to reflect on the significance embedded in this moment of time as we uncover the prophetic meaning woven into each month and season on God's calendar. Together, we will explore the richness of biblical history, the power of spiritual alignment, and the tools for living a life of purpose and promise.

Scripture occasionally uses numbers not merely for counting, but as *theological patterns woven into the fabric of God's revelation*. These patterns are not mystical codes, nor are they meant to predict future events. Rather, they function as *literary and theological signposts* that help God's people recognize recurring themes of covenant, creation, and redemption.

As Dr. Michael S. Heiser frequently cautioned, biblical numerology must remain tethered to clear textual anchors and canonical theology without drifting into speculative or pseudo-mystical systems. Likewise, Dr. G. K. Beale reminds us that such patterns ultimately point to Yeshua, the Temple, and the new creation—not to hidden timelines or secret knowledge.

With that in mind, the Hebrew year 5786 may be read reflectively—not prophetically—by observing the biblical motifs commonly associated with its individual digits: **5**, **7**, **8**, and **6**. Together, these themes form a coherent theological portrait that can shape prayer, discipleship, and communal reflection.

5 I Covenant provision and formative instruction. The number five is most clearly anchored in Scripture through the *Pentateuch*, the five books of *Torah* that form the foundation of Israel's covenant life (Genesis-Deuteronomy). *Torah* is not merely law in a legal sense, but God's gracious instruction—His revealed way of forming a people who reflect His character. Within this *Torah* framework, the sacrificial system is laid out in a structured, deliberate manner (Leviticus 1-7), emphasizing God's provision for atonement, restoration, and communion.

Narratively, the number five often appears in moments of divine sufficiency rather than human strength: David selects five smooth stones before confronting Goliath (1 Samuel 17:40), and Yeshua feeds the multitude with five loaves, demonstrating God's abundance through seemingly inadequate means (John 6:9). Together, these patterns suggest that five carries the weight of *covenant provision, divine sufficiency, and God's gracious instruction for life.*

7 | Divine completeness and covenant fulfillment. If five introduces God's instruction, then seven signals its completion and fulfillment. The seven-day creation account establishes a rhythm in which God brings order, meaning, and rest to the cosmos (Genesis 1:1-2:3). The seventh day—the Sabbath—becomes a covenant sign, reminding Israel that life is sustained not by endless labor, but by trust in God's completed work (Exodus 20:8-11).

Throughout Scripture, and especially in apocalyptic literature, the number seven appears as a marker of divine completeness and intentional design. In Revelation, cycles of seven (e.g., churches, seals, trumpets) communicate God's sovereign orchestration of history toward its appointed end. These sevens are deeply connected to temple imagery and the ultimate restoration of God's dwelling with humanity. Seven, therefore, illustrates *God's faithful completion of His purposes and the wholeness of covenant life under His reign.*

8 | New creation and covenant renewal. Where seven represents completion, eight signals what comes *after* completion—a new beginning. For example, circumcision is commanded on the eighth day as the sign of Abraham's covenant (Genesis 17:12; Leviticus 12:3). This "eighth-day" marker points beyond the natural cycle of a week, symbolizing renewed life and restored identity within God's covenant.

The New Testament expands on this theme by linking circumcision to baptism (Colossians 2:11-12), and baptism to resurrection life (Romans 6:4). Early Christian theology recognized the eighth day as the day of resurrection—the dawn of the new creation inaugurated in Yeshua. Thus, eight consistently represents *renewal, transformation, and life beyond the old order*, rooted not in human effort but in God's redemptive action.

6 | Human vocation and limitation. The number six brings the focus back to humanity's role within God's world. Humanity is created on the sixth day and entrusted with stewardship, responsibility, and work (Genesis 1:26-31).

The covenant pattern of six days of labor followed by Sabbath rest reinforces this vocational rhythm under God's authority (Exodus 20:9).

At the same time, six also illustrates human limitation. In Revelation, the "number of a man" (666) symbolizes humanity exalted apart from God—labor without rest, power without submission, work severed from worship (Revelation 13:18). Thus, the number six holds both dignity and danger: the calling to faithful labor and the reminder that human effort alone cannot bring redemption.

The Hebrew Year of 5786

When read together, the numbers **5+7+8+6** form a theologically rich sequence rather than a mystical code. In this way, the year **5786** may be understood as a season that highlights:

- God's covenantal provision and instruction = **5**,
- moving toward divine completeness and faithful obedience = **7**,
- opening into renewed life in Yeshua = **8**,
- while calling God's people to humble, faithful labor within a still-broken world = **6**.

This reading does not predict events or assign hidden meaning to the Hebrew calendar. Instead, it offers a biblically anchored lens through which God's people can reflect on discipleship, formation, and faithfulness in the present moment.

In keeping with the wisdom of Scripture and the protection of sound scholarship, such patterns invite us to live wisely, obediently, and wholeheartedly with God in the expectant hope of Yeshua's return.

PROLOGUE

The real voyage of discovery consists not in seeking new landscapes, but in having new eyes.

MARCEL PROUST

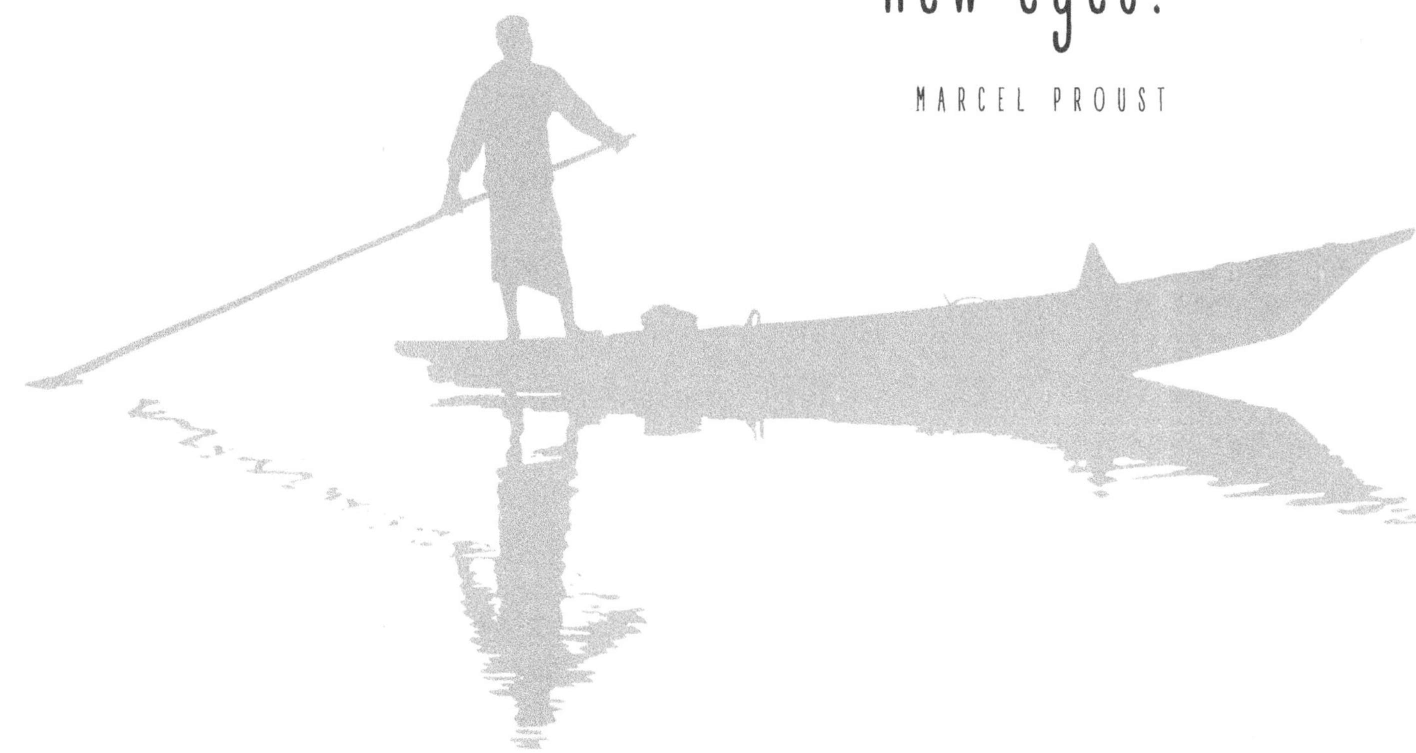

INTRODUCTION

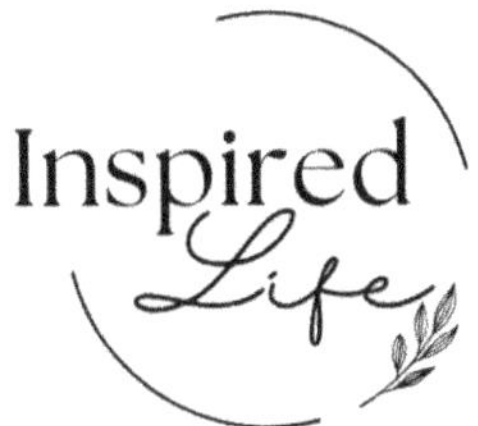

By the grace of God, new beginnings are available to us every moment of every day, but it usually isn't until we hit some sort of marker (like the beginning a new year) that we really appreciate (or even take notice of) the possibilities offered by a fresh start. And this book is just one small part of that process...the first of *many* fresh starts.

> **ROMANS 8:29-30 MSG** | God knew what he was doing from the very beginning. He decided from the outset to shape the lives of those who love him along the same lines as the life of his Son. The Son stands first in the line of humanity he restored. We see the original and intended shape of our lives there in him. After God made that decision of what his children should be like, he followed it up by calling people by name. After he called them by name, he set them on a solid basis with himself. And then, after getting them established, he stayed with them to the end, gloriously completing what he had begun.

We'd like to begin our time together with a confession. We are approaching this year with the assumption that God is *always seeking our transformation through union with Him*. If this assumption is correct, then we are left with two options: (1) put all of our trust Him and align with His purposes OR (2) do it our own way. [Thankfully, I have made enough mistakes over the years to choose the first option].

But if we trust that our union with God will bring transformation, then what does it look like? And how do we align with what He is up to in our lives?

An important aspect of this transformation is described in Isaiah 43:18-19 CJB, where God reminds us to, *"Stop dwelling on past events and brooding over times gone by; I am doing something new; it's springing up — can't you see it? I am making a road in the desert, rivers in the wasteland."*

INTRODUCTION

Freeing ourselves from whatever we are "dwelling on" and "brooding over" starts with (1) naming those things and then, (2) and bringing them to Jesus to be properly grieved. When we choose to live in this freedom, it is easier to attune our heart to the voice of Jesus, the Good Shepherd, who is leading us into God's story for our lives.

This is actually a huge relief. In other words, we no longer have "make life happen" on our own. Instead, we can just listen to our Shepherd's voice and follow where he directs us. Even though we may not always know exactly where we are being led (and we often don't), we do know that *God is deeply and personally committed our restoration...to make us whole and holy* (Ephesians 1:4-6 MSG).

In surrendering ourselves to this process of restoration, we become increasingly aligned with God. In partnership with Him, we experience the comprehensive transformation described in Romans 8:29-30 that unfolds over time. In His great kindness and mercy, *God promises to be with us...but He does not promise that the process will always be easy.* The pain is real...but so is the prize. *And the prize is God Himself.*

So, if this is truly what God is up to...our transformation into wholeness and holiness...then doesn't it just make sense to be as intentional as possible in cultivating our union with Him?

The year 2026 offers renewed hopes and new possibilities, so bring a spirit of expectancy as we map out the year together.

Your dreams are inspired by the deep desires that you were given by the Great Designer...*and these desires point to your destiny.*

Part 1 of *Living An Inspired Life* is an opportunity to consider everything that happened in 2025...and to courageously and intentionally move forward into 2026! This is a priceless investment in yourself!

Setting aside time to reflect on the past twelve months gifts you the opportunity to step into the new year fully empowered to make different choices, learn deeper truths, and embrace new possibilities.

INTRODUCTION

As you use this time to identify both your successes and your sorrows…it will become readily apparent just how much can happen in a year...

...and to truly receive all the possibilities that it brings.

To get the most from this guide, we recommend listening to some relaxing music, pouring yourself a hot beverage, releasing your expectations, and then beginning whenever you're ready.

To complete **Part 1** you will need:

- ❑ At least two hours of uninterrupted time for reflection and planning out the year.
- ❑ A calendar of the past year.
- ❑ A printed version of the *Living An Inspired Life* guide.
- ❑ A selection of your favorite pens.
- ❑ Honesty and openness.

As Søren Kierkegaard reminds us, *"Life can only be understood backwards; but it must be lived forwards."*

However, to fully embrace the story God has written for you also requires *whole-heartedness*, *maturity*, and *courage*…

INTRODUCTION

People often complain about lack of time when lack of direction is the real problem.

ZIG ZIGLAR

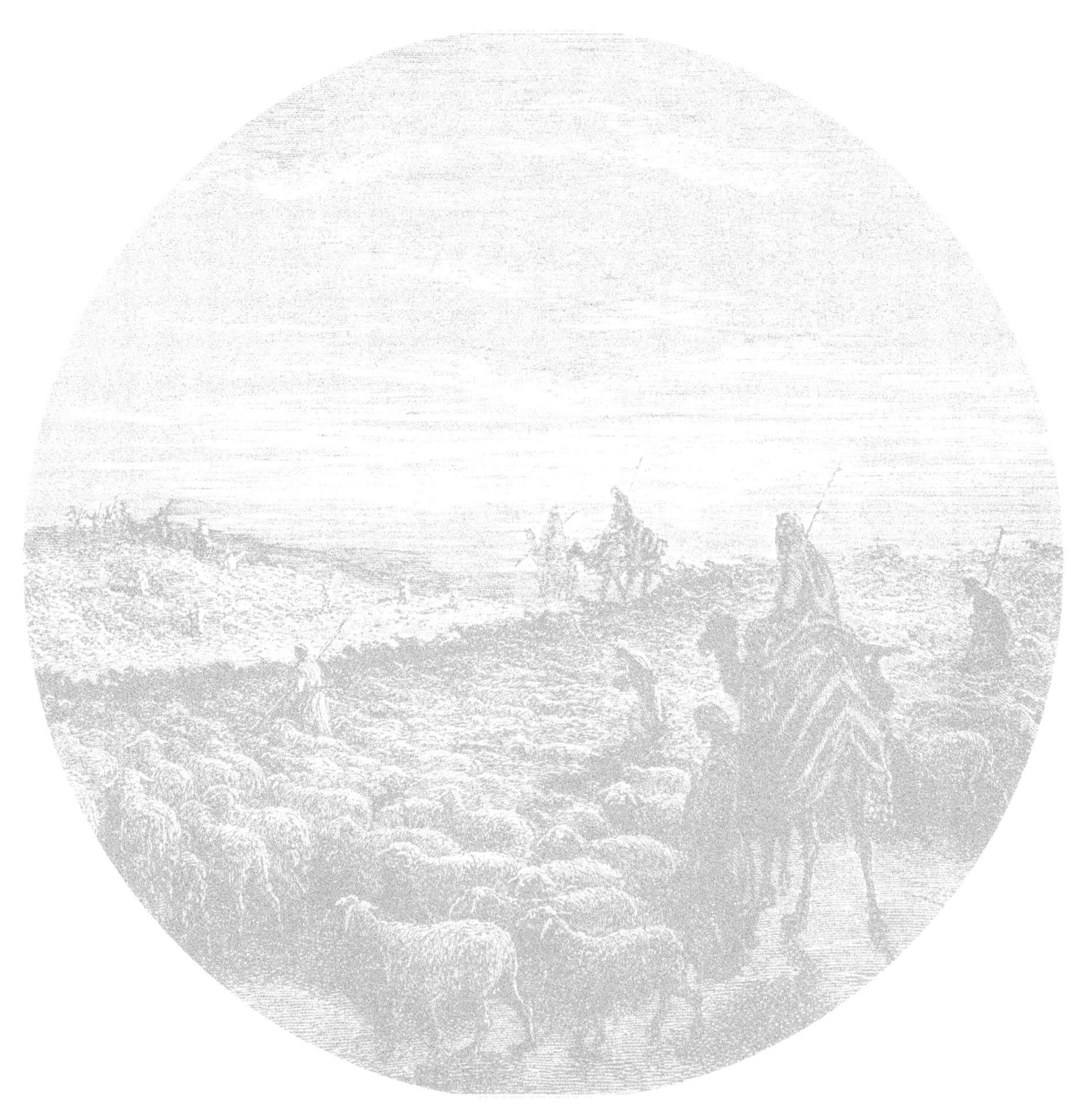

MAPPING YOUR BEST YEAR

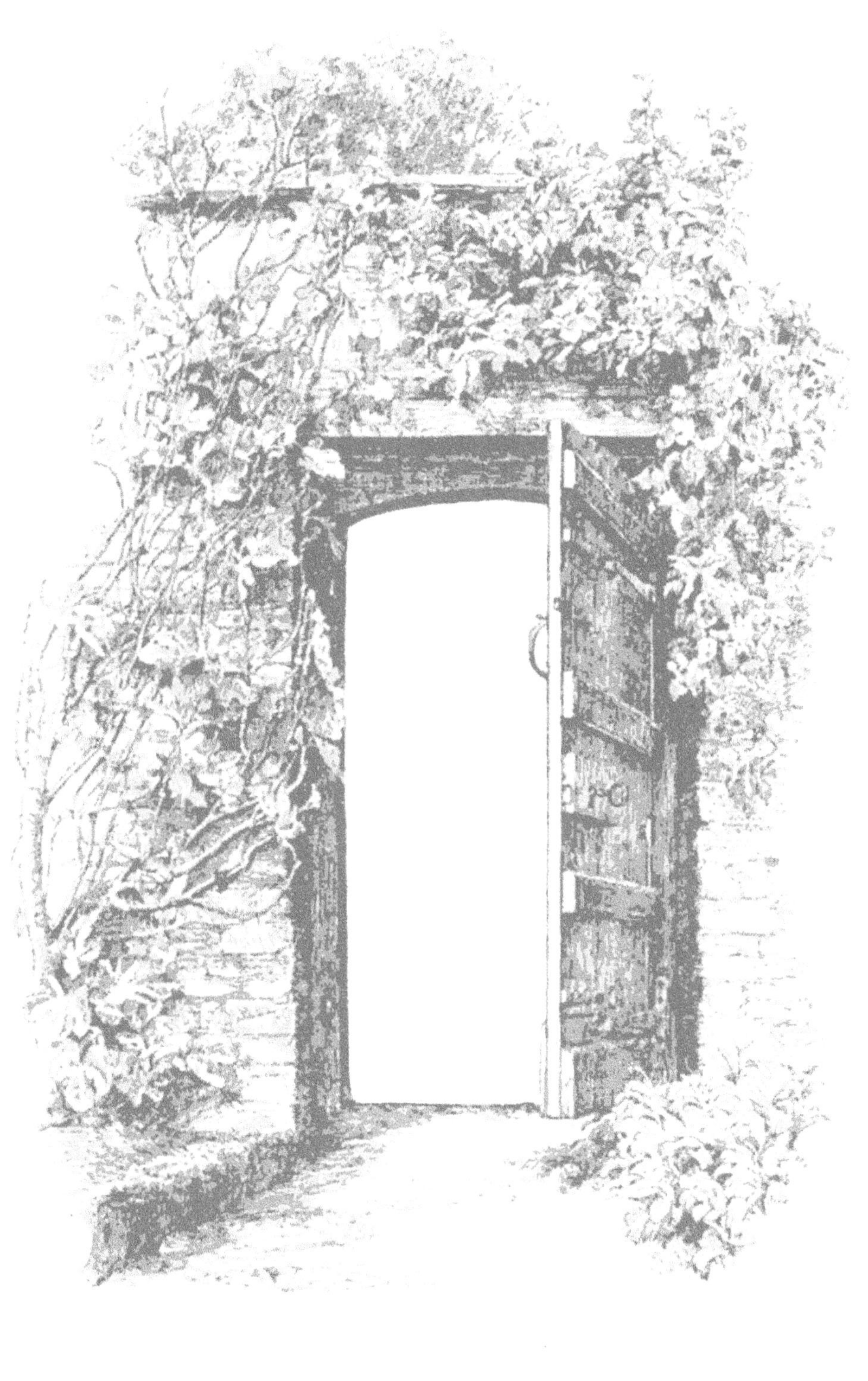

Part 1

MAPPING YOUR BEST YEAR

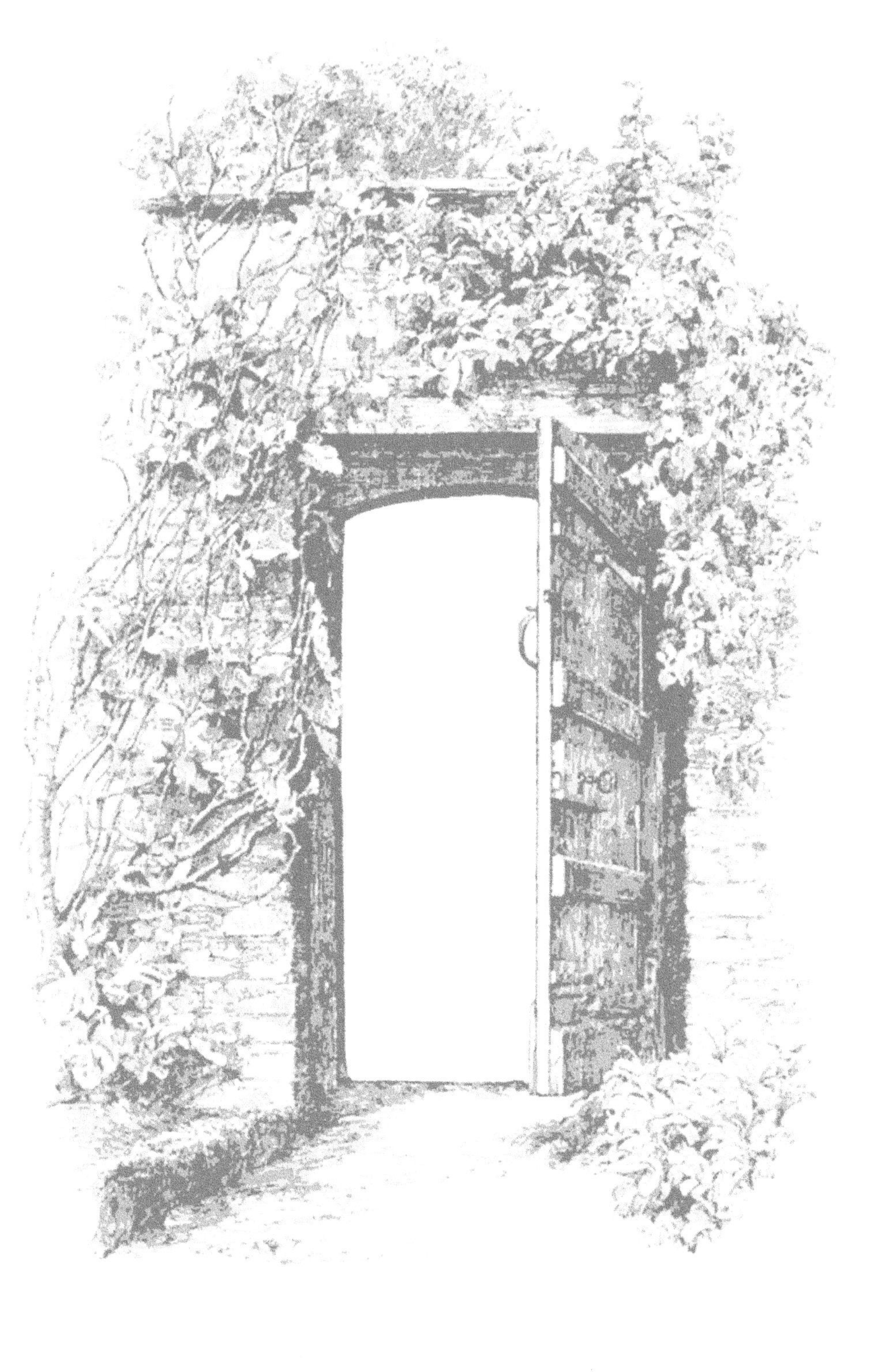

Part 1

YOUR REFLECTION ON THE YEAR

The 2025 Reflection

Before moving into the new year, it's important to first explore the events of this past year and how you were affected by those events.

The year 2025 contained unexpected and unique challenges for all of us but this guide will equip you with tools to process the *spiritual*, *emotional*, and *physical* toll of this past year's events.

These tools focus on three specific areas:

1. **Emotional completion with people/events from the past year.**
2. **Navigating your hopes, dreams, and expectations for the past year.**
3. **Assessing the health of your social circle.**

We will walk with you *every step of the way* as you become complete with the traumas you may have experienced this past year and find peace and resilience amidst the turmoil.

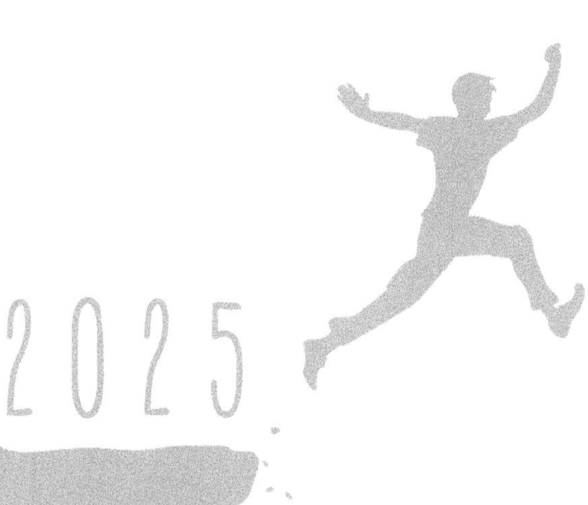

Disclaimer: The year 2025 may have been extremely challenging for you...perhaps you encountered loss, insecurity, or stress. You may find that completing **Part I** of the guide brings up strong feelings, and while we believe it is a powerful tool, it is not a replacement for therapy. If you feel severe or overwhelming emotional discomfort, please seek professional help.

ACTIVITIES: Redefining Control

Although it's easy to believe otherwise, there are really only three things under your control—(1) your *words*, (2) your *actions*, and (3) your *emotional responses*. Everything else is *outside of your power*.

Unfortunately, we often spend much of our time obsessing and worrying about things that we have no real influence over. Let's recalibrate that.

Write down everything that concerns you right now. Then, go back and circle the items you can solve on your own by saying something, doing something, or reframing your emotions.

Whatever is NOT circled are the things you need to surrender. Remind yourself that you don't have to bear the weight of the world on your shoulders. Just concentrate on your own words, actions, and emotions.

Release the rest and surrender it to God.

ACTIVITIES: What Losses Did You Experience This Past Year?

The year 2025 was full of changes, both large and small. We define loss as a change in a familiar pattern of behavior…which can describe events and experiences that we did not previously consider a "loss." Did you experience any transitions this year? (Transitions often bring conflicting emotions).

Write down any losses you have experienced this year.

ACTIVITIES: Emotionally Processing Your Year

If you could express your heart about these losses, what do you wish could have been *different, better or more* about them?

Take a moment to connect to these losses...and then write out your emotional truth by expressing what you wish could have been different, better or more about what you experienced this past year.

YOUR REFLECTION ON THE YEAR

ACTIVITIES: Re-Assess Your Year

It's important to honor your victories. As you connect to your emotional truth concerning the losses you experienced, take a moment to write down anything you did to take care of yourself this past year.

Write these experiences down.

ACTIVITIES: An Even Better Tomorrow

Are there any areas in your life you would like to invite God into deeper healing with?

Write down these areas.

YOUR TRIBE: The Health Of Your Community

Transitions in life can sometimes bring changes to our social circles. In some ways, we are much more affected by lost social connections than lost activities and routines.

Think about the people you either lost touch with or have become disconnected from over the past year. Write down how this made you feel.

YOUR TRIBE: A Smaller Circle

Transitions also impact changes within our relationships. Sometimes this means fewer people, but it can also mean deeper connections and more quality time with each other.

Who are close to you these days? Who did you maintain regular contact with this past year, and how?

YOUR REFLECTION ON THE YEAR

YOUR TRIBE: Is Everyone Present?

Take a look at your present core circle of friends. Are you happy with them? Is there someone you miss or would like to add to your core circle?

YOUR TRIBE: Your Best People

What three people were you closest to this year? What kept you together? What are you most grateful to them for? Consider texting, calling, or sending them a card to let them know.

1.
2.
3.

YOUR TRIBE: Looking Forward

List three things you'll do to keep your existing core circle close.

List things you'll do to reconnect with anyone you miss from your circle.

Summarize & Celebrate

You made it to the end of your reflection on the year. Congratulations!

Every year is different and has its share of both disappointments and victories. So please take a moment to celebrate yourself. You got through a challenging year, and that is no small feat!

Use the remaining space on this page to express everything that you feel about what you accomplished this past year!

YOUR YEAR IN [RE]VIEW

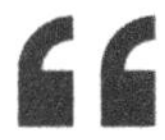

What the new year brings to you will depend a great deal on what you bring to the new year.

Review your 2025 calendar week by week.

Whenever you see an important event, family gathering, friendly get-together, or a significant project, write it down here.

YOUR YEAR IN [RE]VIEW

This Is What 2025 Was About...

Over the past year, which of the following categories were the most important to you? Briefly summarize which events were the most significant.

PERSONAL LIFE & FAMILY

BELONGINGS (HOME, OBJECTS, ETC.)

FRIENDS & COMMUNITY

FINANCES

WORK AND/OR STUDIES

RELAXATION, HOBBIES, CREATIVITY

EMOTIONAL

HEALTH & FITNESS

SPIRITUAL

BUCKET LIST

The Six Best Of 2025

The wisest decision I made…

The biggest lesson I learned…

The biggest risk I took…

The biggest surprise of the year…

The most important thing I did for others…

The biggest thing I completed…

The Six Questions Of 2025

What are you most proud of?

Who are the three people who influenced you the most?

1.
2.
3.

Who are the three people you influenced the most?

1.
2.
3.

What were you not able to accomplish?

What is the best thing you discovered about yourself?

What are you most grateful for?

YOUR YEAR IN [RE]VIEW

The Big Three Of 2025

What were your three greatest accomplishments from last year?

What did you do to achieve these three accomplishments?

Who helped you achieve these successes?

What were your three greatest challenges from last year?

Who or what helped you overcome these challenges?

What have you learned about yourself from overcoming these challenges?

YOUR YEAR IN [RE]VIEW

What word, phrase, or Scripture did God give you for 2025?

What did that word, phrase, or Scripture come to mean to you throughout the year?

What negative belief (concerning God, yourself, other people, or how life works) do you struggle with the most?

Undelivered communication keeps us emotionally incomplete, so writing down your thoughts and feelings will help you finish this year strong and begin the next with a healthy mindset.

Write down anything you want to express about the events of 2024 and say "Goodbye." Are you holding on to unforgiveness for someone? For yourself? Be sure you include the negative belief you wrote down above.

You are done with the past year and emotionally complete with 2025! Now take a deep breath and 2026 here we come...

Dare To Dream Big

As you leave 2025 behind, are you ready to experience everything that God has prepared for the year ahead? It's an important question...and we have personally experienced the power of this simple system.

After incorporating the steps described in the *Living An Inspired Life* guide, you will develop greater clarity into your true desires...and how to live the beautiful story that God has written for your life.

The goals that people set for themselves *often have very little to do with their true desires...and A LOT to do with the expectations of others*. Striving to meet these expectations causes us to feel overwhelmed and allows feelings of failure to infect every part of our lives. It's also why so many people fail to achieve their goals...and often feel unfulfilled by the ones they do achieve.

Goals CAN be productive IF they are supported by (1) *God's direction* and (2) *an achievable, concrete plan of action*. This is the difference between just setting goals and really connecting to what makes us feel alive!

What excites you about the next 12 months?

Review the negative beliefs you just released...what is the TRUTH you will replace it with as you live out the next 12 months?

YOUR YEAR IN [PRE]VIEW

This Is What My Next Year Will Be About...

Number the following categories in order of importance for 2026 and briefly summarize their significance to you.

PERSONAL LIFE & FAMILY

BELONGINGS (HOME, OBJECTS, ETC.)

FRIENDS & COMMUNITY

FINANCES

WORK AND/OR STUDIES

RELAXATION, HOBBIES, CREATIVITY

EMOTIONAL

HEALTH & FITNESS

SPIRITUAL

BUCKET LIST

The Big Three Of 2026

What are three things you WILL choose to love about yourself?

What are three things you WILL choose to let go of?

What are the three things you most want to achieve in 2025?

List the three people who are your biggest supporters.

1.

2.

3.

What are three things you WILL regularly choose to do to encourage yourself?

What are three things you WILL commit to doing every day?

Things On My Heart For 2026

I want to connect with my loved ones in these ways…

This is what I most want to communicate to my loved ones…

These are the places I want to visit…

This year, I will no longer procrastinate about…

This year, I will intentionally invest in this particular relationship…

This is the ONE thing I REALLY want to happen this year (and why)…

The Year Ahead

Has God given you a word, phrase, or Scripture for 2026? Write it down.

Write down anything that comes to mind about that word, phrase, or Scripture.

Unleash your heart...what is your secret wish for 2026?

Congratulations…you are done planning the year ahead! By choosing to be intentional about 2026, you just made a great investment in yourself, and we stand with you in the belief that anything is possible for this year!

If you have built castles in the air, your work need not be lost; that is where they should be. Now put the foundations under them.

HENRY DAVID THOREAU

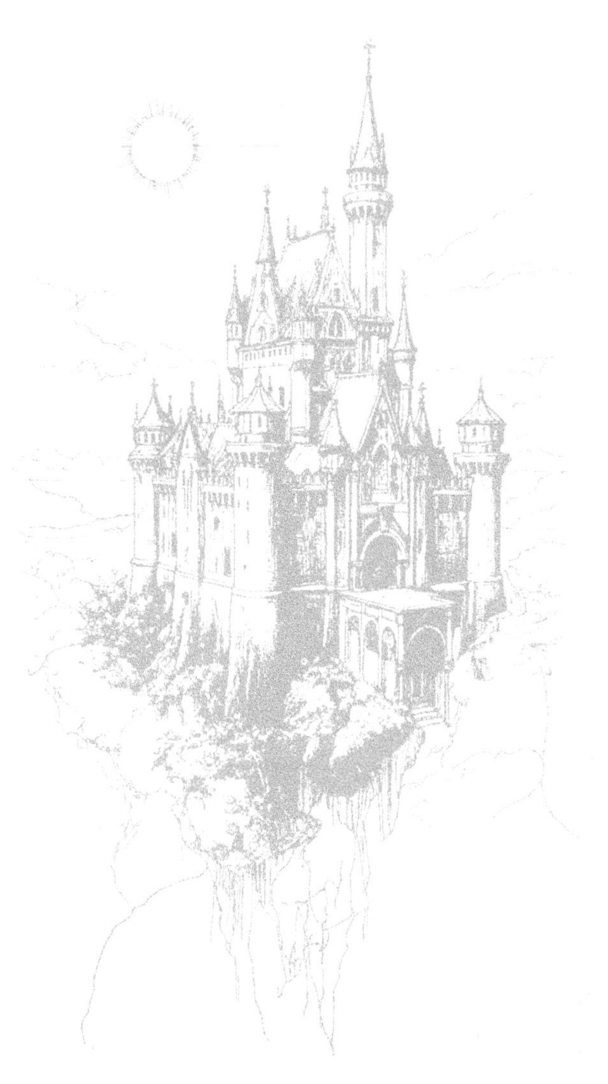

ALIGNING WITH GOD'S DESIGN

We believe that God created our lives with meaning and purpose...but how does it all work? Since He exists outside of time, God enters our future to speak the necessary Word to empower us to live the story that He has written for our lives. (Psalm 139:16)

But do you *trust* God's design and destiny for your life?

Every season of life offers the promise of healing and growth...but it does not "just happen." To that end, God partners with us to bring about the fulfillment of His promises. So, are you ready to receive what He has promised?

Your desire reveals your design, and your design reveals your destiny...

What are you passionate about? What has God placed on your heart?

However, since our destiny is ruthlessly contested by the Adversary, it is essential to rely on God's strength for the fight...*and half our battles are won during worship.* In those moments of intense conflict, God is drawing us into agreement with what He has spoken over our lives. It is time to declare...

"I will only *believe* what God says and will *entertain* no other voices. I am a *warrior* who draws strength from what He speaks over my life. I rely on the Word of God to interpret and overcome the obstacles blocking my path."

1 TIMOTHY 1:18-19 TPT | So Timothy, my son, I [Paul] am entrusting you with this responsibility, in keeping with the very first prophecies that were spoken over your life and are now in the process of fulfillment in this great work of ministry, in keeping with the prophecies spoken over you. With this encouragement use your prophecies as weapons as you wage spiritual warfare by faith and with a clean conscience.

ALIGNING WITH GOD'S DESIGN

Each year brings the opportunity to partner with God to declare the story that *He has entrusted you with.*

It is interesting to note that the decade of the 20's is aligned with the Hebrew decade of the 80's through its connection to the Hebrew letter "*Pei.*" *Pei* symbolizes the mouth and represents the decade of speaking and declaring. *When your words align with the words God is speaking over your life, it forms a double-edged sword that nothing in all creation can stand against.*

You are not defined by your past. Your past is not your destiny. Your destiny is established by God...we just strive to remain in alignment with what He has already declared! (Psalm 139:16)

We *can* choose to live in great expectancy of what God has planned for us.

When you stand in agreement with God over your calling, your career, and your sphere of influence; He will give you clarity, insight, and blessing.

The path to thriving is found through aligning ourselves with God's design.

> "By doing what His Word and His Spirit tell us to do, giving Him the sacrifice of worship and staying in the glory of His presence no matter what is happening around us, we will be rightly aligned and positioned for advancement in His time.
>
> CHUCK D. PIERCE

This alignment is experienced within the three foundational elements of human existence...*Spirit...Mind...Body.*

We will begin with the Spirit because He is the ultimate source of power for everything else. Take some time with each of the following questions and write down ways you can be intentional in each of these three areas of your life.

> "This is living a life by design, not default...and this is how we thrive.
>
> GET INSPIRED MOVEMENT

ALIGNING WITH GOD'S DESIGN

What do you want your personal connection with God to be like this year?

What is one thing you will do this year to step into God's design for your life?

SPIRIT

Who will you seek mentorship from? Who will you seek to mentor? What will that look like?

SPIRIT

ALIGNING WITH GOD'S DESIGN

What will I learn (e.g., personal growth, education, books I want to read, etc.)?

MIND

How will I steward my finances (e.g., savings, investments, debt elimination)?

MIND

How will I live out my passions (e.g., travel, dreams, talents, projects)?

MIND

ALIGNING WITH GOD'S DESIGN

Food...How will I eat in healthy, balanced moderation?

BODY

Exercise...What will I do to be consistent in exercise?

BODY

Health...How will I invest in my health (e.g., massage, supplements, chiropractic adjustments, etc.)?

BODY

A map does more than mark distances and directions…it unveils meaning. It teaches us how to see where we are, and in doing so, discloses unsuspected connections—bridges between here and there, between truths that had long stood apart, waiting to be recognized as belonging to the same landscape.

UNKNOWN

THE ALIGNMENT MAP

Once you have *grieved* and *celebrated* the previous year...it is time to begin thinking through what you would like to see happen this year...

This is the perfect time to take concrete steps toward aligning with everything that God intends for the year ahead.

STEP NO. 1: Start by writing down every desire that you have for the new year. No wish is too small or too large. Give your imagination full permission to run wild.

STEP NO. 2: Set aside some time, find a quiet place where you feel comfortable, and pray through each one of the desires you wrote down. God might reveal that you didn't dream big enough. He might show you that your desires will lead you away from His intended best. Or He might simply tell you, "Yes, but not yet." Just be open to receiving whatever He says.

1 CHRONICLES 16:11 CJB | [11] Seek ADONAI and his strength; always seek his presence.

MATTHEW 26:39, 42, 44 CJB | [39] Going on a little farther, he [Yeshua] fell on his face, praying, "My Father, if possible, let this cup pass from me! Yet — *not what I want, but what you want!*" [...] [42] A second time he went off and prayed. "My Father, if this cup cannot pass away unless I drink it, *let what you want be done*." [...] [44] Leaving them again, he went off and prayed a third time, *saying the same words*.

JOHN 16:4 CJB | [4] Till now you haven't asked for anything in my [Yeshua's] name. Keep asking, and you will receive, so that your joy may be complete.

PHILIPPIANS 4:6 CJB | [6] Don't worry about anything; on the contrary, make your requests known to God by prayer and petition, with thanksgiving.

We live our best lives when our talents, passions, and desires fully align with God's purposes. This alignment empowers us to move forward with confidence into union with Him. After praying through each of your desires, write down any insights that God shares with you.

____

____

____

____

____

THE ALIGNMENT MAP

STEP NO. 3: This is where we translate alignment into action. Set aside 20-30 uninterrupted minutes for this exercise.

Choose your focus. Review the desires you reflected on in **STEP NO. 2**. From that list, *select one to three desires that feel*:

- Energizing rather than draining.
- Realistic for the next year.
- Aligned with your talents, interests, and current capacity.

These are not "someday" ideas. They are priorities for the year ahead. *Write your selected desires below*:

(1) ______________________________

(2) ______________________________

(3) ______________________________

Define a clear outcome. For each desire, describe one specific outcome you would like to see by the end of the year. *Ask yourself, "How will I know this desire has been meaningfully expressed?"*:

Desired Outcome No. 1: ______________________________

____

Desired Outcome No. 2: ______________________________

____

Desired Outcome No. 3: ______________________________

____

Identify the next right actions. For each outcome, list *two or three practical actions you can take in the next 90 days*. Keep these actions:

- Small enough to realistically schedule.
- Concrete enough to reasonably complete.
- Focused on progress, not perfection.

Desired Outcome No. 1 | 90-Day Actions: ______________________________

____

____

____

Desired Outcome No. 2 | 90-Day Actions: ______________________________

____

____

____

Desired Outcome No. 3 | 90-Day Actions: ______________________________

____

____

____

Anticipate and prepare. Consider one likely *obstacle* for each desire and *your response*. *This is not pessimism—it is preparation*.

THE ALIGNMENT MAP

Desired Outcome No. 1 | Obstacle: ______________________________

____

Response: ______________________________

____

Desired Outcome No. 2 | Obstacle: ______________________________

____

Response: ______________________________

____

Desired Outcome No. 3 | Obstacle: ______________________________

____

Response: ______________________________

____

Reflection. Alignment isn't created through pressure—it's sustained through intention. When your actions reflect your talents, passions, and clarified desires, confidence grows naturally, and forward movement becomes steadier and more meaningful.

STEP NO. 4: Be committed to (daily) alignment with God and with who He says you are to remain anchored in His Truth. Review the following forty Scriptures that declare the "truest truth" about who we are in God's love (as often as needed). ☺

1. I AM SAVED

2 TIMOTHY 1:9 CJB | 9 since he [Yeshua] delivered us and called us to a life of holiness as his people. It was not because of our deeds, but because of his own purpose and the grace which he gave to us who are united with the Messiah Yeshua. He did this before the beginning of time, [...]

2. I AM COMPLETE

COLOSSIANS 2:10 CJB | 10 And it is in union with him that you have been made full — he is the head of every rule and authority.

3. I AM CHOSEN

1 THESSALONIANS 1:4 CJB | 4 We know, brothers, that God has loved and chosen you;

4. I AM FORGIVEN

1 JOHN 2:12 CJB | 12 You children, I am writing you because your sins have been forgiven for his sake.

5. I AM A NEW CREATION

2 CORINTHIANS 5:17 CJB | 17 Therefore, if anyone is united with the Messiah, he is a new creation — the old has passed; look, what has come is fresh and new!

6. I AM A CHILD OF GOD

1 JOHN 3:1 CJB | 3 See what love the Father has lavished on us in letting us be called God's children! For that is what we are. The reason the world does not know us is that it has not known him.

7. I AM REDEEMED

EPHESIANS 1:7-8 CJB | [7] In union with him, through the shedding of his blood, we are set free — our sins are forgiven; this accords with the wealth of the grace [8] he has lavished on us.

8. I AM LIGHT

MATTHEW 5:14 CJB | [14] "You are light for the world. A town built on a hill cannot be hidden."

9. I AM JUSTIFIED

ROMANS 5:1 CJB | [5] So, since we have come to be considered righteous by God because of our trust, let us continue to have shalom [peace] with God through our Lord, Yeshua the Messiah.

10. I AM FREE FROM SIN

ROMANS 6:22 CJB | [22] However, now, freed from sin and enslaved to God, you do get the benefit — it consists in being made holy, set apart for God, and its end result is eternal life.

11. I AM A SUPERCONQUEROR

ROMANS 8:37 CJB | [37] No, in all these things we are superconquerors, through the one who has loved us.

12. I AM GOD'S TEMPLE

1 CORINTHIANS 3:16 CJB | [16] Don't you know that you people are God's temple and that God's Spirit lives in you?

13. I AM ONE WITH YESHUA

1 CORINTHIANS 6:17 CJB | [17] but the person who is joined to the Lord is one spirit.

14. I AM CALLED

1 CORINTHIANS 7:17 CJB | [17] Only let each person live the life the Lord has assigned him and live it in the condition he was in when God called him. This is the rule I lay down in all the congregations.

15. I AM CREATED FOR GOOD WORKS

EPHESIANS 2:10 CJB | [10] For we are of God's making, created in union with the Messiah Yeshua for a life of good actions already prepared by God for us to do.

16. I AM SECURE IN YESHUA

COLOSSIANS 3:3 CJB | [3] For you have died, and your life is hidden with the Messiah in God.

17. I AM VICTORIOUS

1 CORINTHIANS 15:57 CJB | [...] [57] but thanks be to God, who gives us the victory through our Lord Yeshua the Messiah!

18. I AM NOT CONDEMNED

ROMANS 8:1 CJB | [1] Therefore, there is no longer any condemnation awaiting those who are in union with the Messiah Yeshua.

19. I AM SAFE

PHILIPPIANS 4:7 CJB | [7] Then God's shalom [peace], passing all understanding, will keep your hearts and minds safe in union with the Messiah Yeshua.

20. I AM AN HEIR

GALATIANS 4:7 CJB | [7] So through God you are no longer a slave but a son, and if you are a son, you are also an heir.

21. I AM ACCEPTED

ROMANS 15:7 CJB | [7] So welcome each other, just as the Messiah has welcomed you into God's glory.

22. I AM AN AMBASSADOR

2 CORINTHIANS 5:20 CJB | [20] Therefore we are ambassadors of the Messiah; in effect, God is making his appeal through us. What we do is appeal on behalf of the Messiah, "Be reconciled to God!"

23. I AM HEALED

PSALM 30:3 CJB | [3] ADONAI my God, I cried out to you, and you provided healing for me.

24. I AM SURROUNDED BY GOD'S GRACE

PSALM 32:10 CJB | [10] Many are the torments of the wicked, but grace surrounds those who trust in ADONAI.

25. I AM SECURE

PSALM 1:3 CJB | [3] They are like trees planted by streams — they bear their fruit in season, their leaves never wither, everything they do succeeds.

26. I AM WONDERFULLY MADE

PSALM 139:14 CJB | [14] I thank you because I am awesomely made, wonderfully; your works are wonders — I know this very well.

27. I AM NOT ALONE

ISAIAH 41:10 CJB | [10] Don't be afraid, for I am with you; don't be distressed, for I am your God. I give you strength, I give you help, I support you with my victorious right hand.

28. I AM AMONG GOD'S PEOPLE

REVELATION 21:3 CJB | [3] I heard a loud voice from the throne say, "See! God's Sh'khinah [Glory] is with mankind, and he will live with them. They will be his people, and he himself, God-with-them, will be their God.

29. I AM STRONG

2 CORINTHIANS 12:10 CJB | [10] Yes, I am well pleased with weaknesses, insults, hardships, persecutions, and difficulties endured on behalf of the Messiah; for it is when I am weak that I am strong.

30. I AM BLESSED

PSALM 84:5 CJB | [5] How happy are those who live in your house; they never cease to praise you!

31. I AM SPECIAL TO GOD

1 PETER 2:9 CJB | [9] But you are a chosen people, the King's Cohanim [priests], a holy nation, a people for God to possess! Why? In order for you to declare the praises of the One who called you out of darkness into his wonderful light.

32. I AM FULLY ALIVE

EPHESIANS 2:4-5 CJB | [4] But God is so rich in mercy and loves us with such intense love [5] that, even when we were dead because of our acts of disobedience, he brought us to life along with the Messiah — it is by grace that you have been delivered.

33. I AM JOYFUL

ROMANS 15:13 CJB | [13] May God, the source of hope, fill you completely with joy and shalom [peace] as you continue trusting, so that by the power of the Ruach HaKodesh [Holy Spirit] you may overflow with hope.

34. I AM COMPETENT

2 CORINTHIANS 3:5 CJB | [5] It is not that we are competent in ourselves to count anything as having come from us; on the contrary, our competence is from God.

35. I AM VALUED

ISAIAH 43:4 CJB | [4] Because I regard you as valued and honored, and because I love you. For you I will give people, nations in exchange for your life.

36. I AM A CITIZEN OF HEAVEN

PHILIPPIANS 3:20 CJB | [20] But we are citizens of heaven, and it is from there that we expect a Deliverer, the Lord Yeshua the Messiah.

37. I AM WONDERFULLY MADE

PSALM 139:14 CJB | [14] I thank you because I am awesomely made, wonderfully; your works are wonders — I know this very well.

38. I AM HOPEFUL

ISAIAH 40:31 CJB | 31 But those who hope in the LORD will renew their strength. They will soar on wings like eagles; they will run and not grow weary; they will walk and not be faint.

39. I AM NOT AFRAID

ISAIAH 43:1 CJB | [43] But now this is what ADONAI says, he who created you, Ya'akov [Jacob], he who formed you, Isra'el: "Don't be afraid, for I have redeemed you; I am calling you by your name; you are mine."

40. I AM WISE IN GOD'S WISDOM

PROVERBS 2:6 CJB | [6] For ADONAI gives wisdom; from his mouth comes knowledge and understanding.

Why Is It So Difficult To Manage Our Time? What Are We Missing?

GALATIANS 5:25 CJB | 25 Since it is through the Spirit that we have Life; let it also be through the Spirit that we *order our lives day by day*.

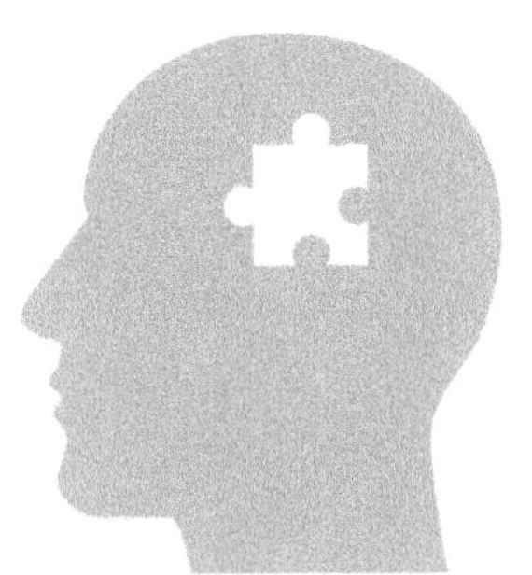

The reason we find managing our time so challenging is probably not the reason most people think. [Yes…the struggle to create a schedule that organizes our lives and efficiently manages our time IS REAL…but there's more to it than just that. A lot more]. *So, why does it feel like there is never enough time in the day*?

I'm going to suggest a couple of things. First, we're using the wrong "ruler" to measure how we use our time. And second, we assume that the failure to complete everything on our never-ending to-do-lists means that we're terrible at scheduling, organizing, and managing time.

But the answer is not that simple and it's definitely incomplete. How else can you explain why our lives seem jam-packed with busyness… *and yet it so often feels like we're not getting anything done*?

Imagine for a moment that you spent every day doing what truly mattered most to you. Even if your life was totally busy, would you still believe that you were terrible at managing time? Probably not. We'll come back to that.

To be perfectly honest with you, I'm not a scheduling guru. I've never been interviewed on national media to discuss my *New York Times* best-selling book on organizational skills. (I haven't published one, by the way). And I don't have a thousand tasks on my "to-do list" that I effortlessly check off each and every day.

But I am absolutely crystal clear about what matters most to our family.

And that's why, more often than not, the *immediate does not interfere with the important.* Trust me, it makes ALL the difference.

I learned (the hard way) that it's not about how many things you get done...it's whether those things you get done really matter. *Better to accomplish one goal that truly matters than 100 that don't.*

So, going forward, I'm defining "time management" as *the intentional use of time to accomplish whatever is most important to us.*

Start By Unlearning What We've Learned

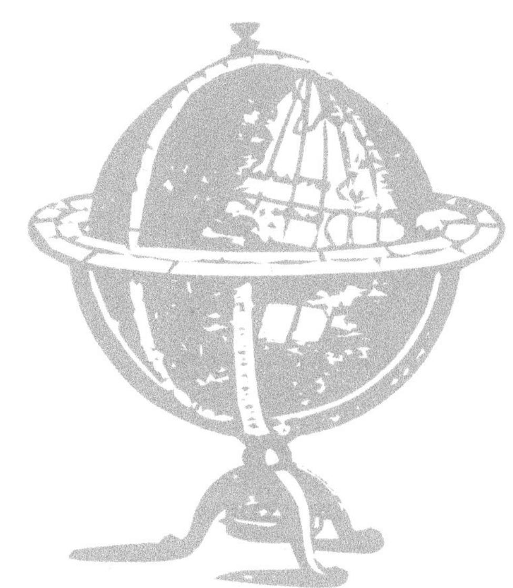

Everyone on planet earth has the same 24-hours every day...but not everyone is intentional about what they do with those hours. Are we truly prioritizing the use of our time? Or are we "at the mercy" of a schedule that's not even our own? If so, why?

Our schooling trained us to believe that everyone learns the *same* things, the *same* way, at the *same* time, at the *same* pace. We were trained to measure good...bad...right...wrong... gifted...lazy...according to whether we finished an arbitrary amount of work within an equally arbitrary amount of time. We were told that our "success" or "failure" depended upon it. Sadly, many of us still believe this lie.

That's why (usually right after New Years) we resolve to re-structure and re-organize our entire lives to become better managers of time so that we can "get more done." And we desperately hope that this new resolution will be our ticket into the "Promised Land" of living a productive life. How's that working out for you?

Me neither.

Unfortunately, many of us compensate for our time-management "failures" by compiling a massive list of goals...which ultimately just sets us up for more failure. That's because when we don't achieve these unrealistic objectives, we just take on the additional burdens of fear, insecurity, shame, or despair.

The Key Is Intentionality

Time will either *promote* you...or *expose* you. So, remember that the "goal of goals" is always *improvement, not perfection*. Therefore, if a goal does not serve you, then it's no longer a goal...*it's a burden.*

Basically, there are two types of goals: (1) "Must-Do" and (2) "Like-To-Do"...*and knowing the difference will make your life much simpler.*

1. Must-Do

In order to qualify for placement on the "Must-Do" list, the goal must be both *essential* and *reasonable.*

How do I know if this goal is this essential?

Ask yourself this question: *"Will achieving this goal still matter ten years from now?"* Your answer will narrow things down considerably and help clarify what is truly important to you.

For example, let's say that your child was supposed to read three chapters of Shakespeare, and they had...um...a "less-than positive" attitude about the assignment. What's more important? Pressing on and forcing them to complete the reading? Or dealing with the reasons behind their resistance? Fast-forward ten years from now...*what do you think will matter more*? That they read Act II of *King Lear*, or that they are a young man or woman with good character? After all, you can spend a little time to address the issue now...or spend A LOT more time band-aiding the situation over several years.

I'm going to suggest that whatever deepens our union with God...whatever brings us into closer alignment with His story for our lives...is *always* a WIN.

How do I know if this goal is reasonable?

In order to determine what is "reasonable" for ourselves...we must take a fearless moral and *non-shaming* inventory of our present situation.

Unrealistic goals are really just future disappointments. While there is nothing wrong with short-term goals (they are often necessary for the achievement of our long-term goals) *your primary concern here is the enduring importance of the goal itself.*

2. Like-To-Do

These are simply things that "would be nice" to accomplish but are non-essential. In other words, they are the icing, not the cake.

NOTE: It's really crucial to avoid treating the goals on your "Like-To-Do" list as essential...it will only confuse and frustrate you.

Goals Do NOT = Commands

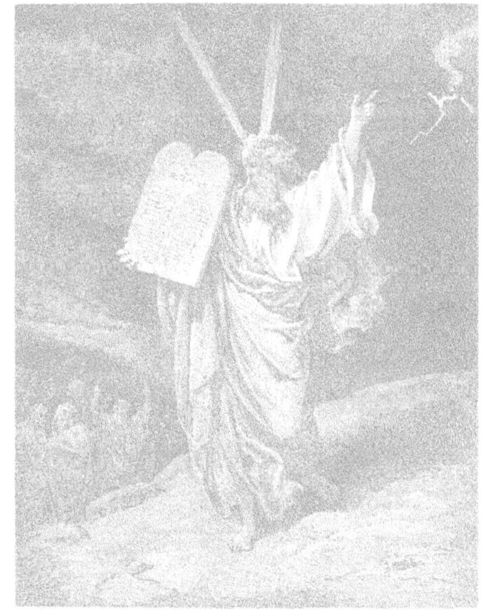

While we can all agree that it's important to have goals [insert "aim at nothing, hit nothing" cliché], remember that they simply measure whether we got the "win." A goal should be regarded as a worthy objective, not a commandment written in stone, "Thou shalt successfully completeth all thy goals or thou art doomed to failure."

The *only* thing that matters is *diligence and excellence of effort*...since the goal of all goals is to partner with God in aligning with His plan to experience everything that He has intended for our lives.

Practice Makes Progress

So, assuming that you did your best that day...*it's always a win*. But if you didn't, instead of booking a guilt trip on Expedia.com®, set aside some time to pray and figure out *why* you didn't bring your best...and try again tomorrow.

And then, just commit yourself to keep on trying.

Decide to "give up on giving up" and keep going whenever you fall short. At the end of the day, what matters most is the *quality of the effort, not the result.* However, if consistently practiced, excellence of effort *will* produce results.

And until it does, you won't run out of God's grace (trust me).

Mapping Out A Plan That Works For You

We all have our own unique rhythms that need to be aligned with God's. So, while there are certain principles (i.e., there is a way that things work), only you and God know the best way to apply those principles when it comes to organizing, scheduling, and managing your time. This is also why "practicals" that may seem to work so well for others, *are not necessarily helpful for you*.

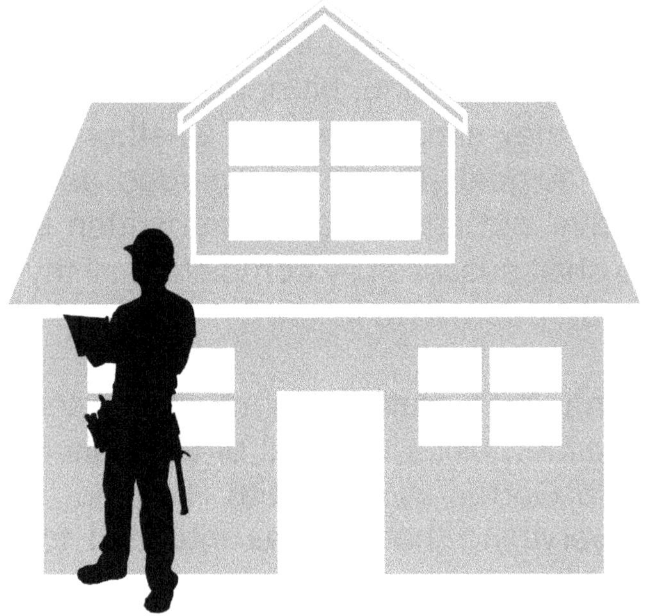

It's a lot like remodeling a house. You have to replace rotten boards and damaged drywall. Then, you have to putty, sand, primer, and paint all the surfaces. But HOW those tasks are accomplished, and the TIME required to complete them is entirely up to you. As long as you're putting forth your best effort to finish the house...what matters most is aligning with God's timing...not how fast the "remodeling" is completed.

The Power Of Reverse-Engineering

It should be noted that the templates provided here are *just suggestions.* But as Paul says, "run your lives by the Spirit" (Galatians 5:16 CJB) and ask God to show you how to align your desires with His purposes for the months and seasons ahead. To that end, we will begin by mapping out your *yearly goals. This is everything you have completed to this point (pp. 2-33) comes together.*

Yearly Goals relate to your spiritual, emotional, mental, social, and physical development...and they represent your most important values and priorities.

Taking the time to *partner with God* in mapping out these goals will help you:

- ❑ **Keep an eye on the big picture.** Setting yearly priorities enables you to stay focused on the *important vs. the immediate*. Our attention exists in conflict between things that are immediate and things that are important...and far too often, the immediate wins.

- ❑ **Unlearn the bad and learn the good.** School indoctrinated us with the false belief that everyone learns the same things, the same way, at the same time, at the same pace. Therefore, ignore humanistic and arbitrary measurements and instead, rely on God's wisdom to set your priorities.

- ❑ **Make your day-to-day life manageable.** When goals are clearly organized into smaller, more easily completable tasks...accomplishing your **Yearly Goals** becomes legitimately doable. By just focusing on the mini-goal for the week, the goals for each month almost happen by themselves (well, not exactly, but you know what I mean). ☺

- ❑ **Gain and maintain momentum.** When the rhythm of your daily actions are aligned with your goals, the confidence that results from consistent accomplishment eventually becomes self-sustaining.

Seeing How It All Works

After carefully praying through each of your twelve **Yearly Goals**...assign one goal to each month (JANUARY thru DECEMBER, pp. 49-64). Then, reverse-engineer how you will achieve each **Monthly Goal** by dividing it into four smaller steps...and then assign those steps to each week of that particular month.

NOTE: There is nothing "magical" about the number twelve. God might prompt you to increase or decrease the number of goals you set. Just make sure that the goal is essential + reasonable + "accomplishable." And some of your goals will likely be on-going…after all, character, like Rome, was not built in a day.

After you've divided your monthly goals into smaller manageable weekly mini-goals, set aside some time each week to review them. If you were unable to accomplish your **Weekly Mini-Goal**…don't worry. Seriously. Cut yourself some slack. BUT it is important to think through WHY you fell short of the mark…

- Were the goals unrealistic? *Renegotiate them.*
- Were the goals realistic, but just needed to be scaled back? *Adjust them.*
- Were you on track to meeting your goals until prevented by an unusual or unexpected circumstance? *Just keep going.*

Talk to God and ask Him for the wisdom to make the necessary adjustments.

By the end of the year, even if you haven't achieved all of your original yearly goals…*you WILL have accomplished the ones that mattered most.*

Remember that time promotes you…or exposes you. So, don't wait for things to get easier, simpler, or better. Life will always be complicated. Learn to be intentional right now. Otherwise, you'll run out of time.

Partner with God to figure out what a "win" for your life looks like…and celebrate every one of them.

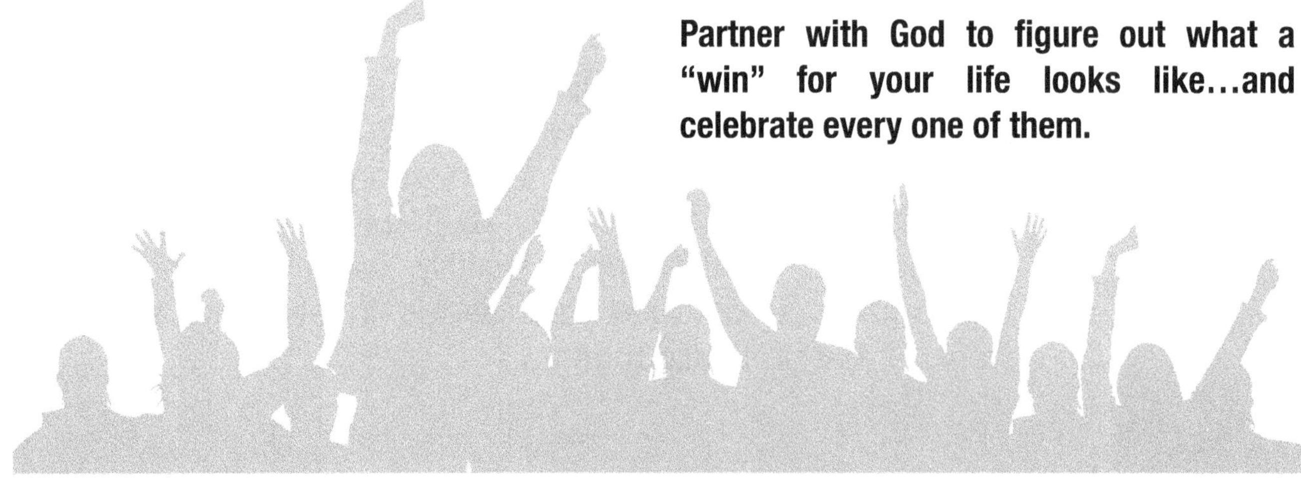

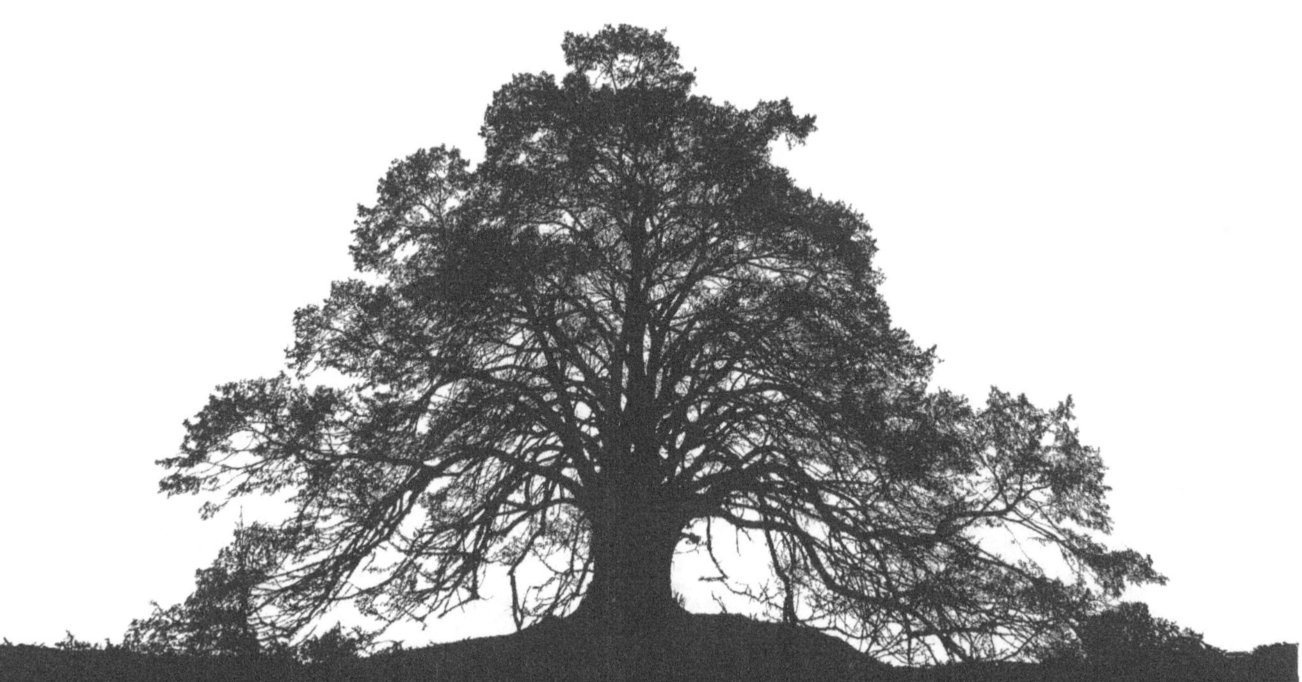

> No amount of money ever bought a second of time.
> UNKNOWN

> I never lose. I either win, or I learn.
> NELSON MANDELA (1918-2013)

Ultimately, goal-setting, scheduling, organizing, and time management…begins by bringing everything under God's authority and then prioritizing the things that are most important. If you commit to building your life around the essential…God, family, friends, and your calling…then even when falling short, you can look forward with confidence, instead of looking back with regret.

There are also foundational truths that shape our goals:

…Our core value as a human being is grounded in our relationship with God.

…Our accomplishments are measured by diligence and excellence of effort, NOT by how far "ahead" or "behind" we are in comparison to others.

…Our happiness is better than wealth…to know the value of things…and not just their price.

THE ALIGNMENT MAP

> Ordinary people think merely of spending time, great people think of using it.
> ARTHUR SCHOPENAUER

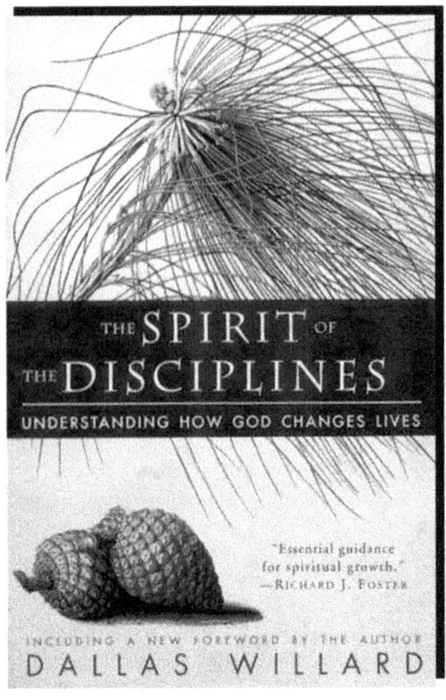

The Spirit of the Disciplines
DALLAS WILLARD

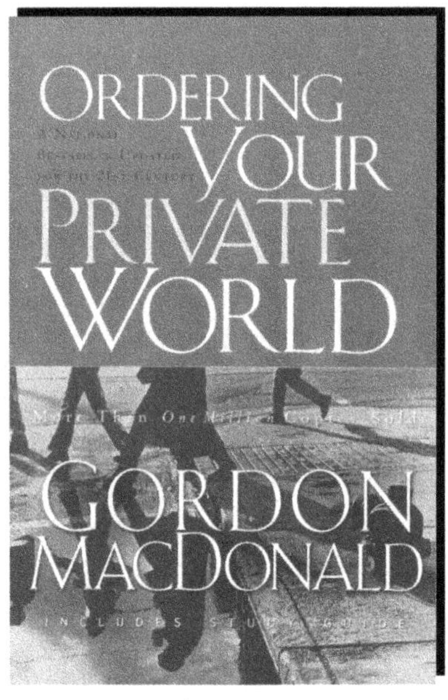

Ordering Your Private World
GORDON MACDONALD

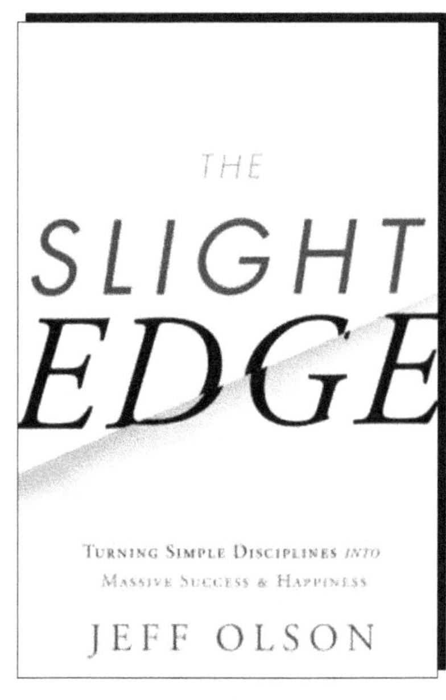

The Slight Edge
JEFF OLSON

[NOTE: As highly as I recommend these resources...they still need to be adapted to what makes sense for where God is leading YOU].

This is where everything you have done to this point all comes together into your partnership with God to create a single roadmap for the year ahead

As a quick review:

- ❑ Carefully pray through each of your twelve **Yearly Goals.**
- ❑ Assign one goal to each month (JANUARY thru DECEMBER, pp. 49-64).
- ❑ Reverse-engineer how you will achieve each **Monthly Goal** by dividing it into four smaller steps.
- ❑ Assign those smaller steps to each week of that particular month.

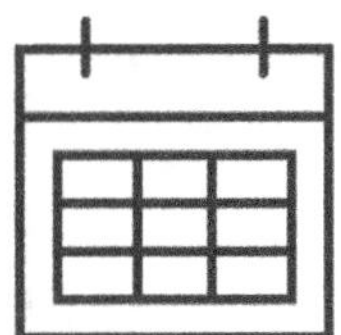

WINS FOR THE YEAR

THE ESSENTIALS

WINTER

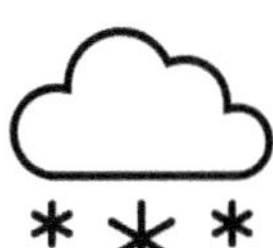

Winter is cold and dreary, and we usually spend most of our time indoors. If Spring is a time for "birthing" then Winter is a time for "conceiving." In other words, we consider the lessons from previous seasons as we partner with God to make plans for moving forward. "The more *reflective* you are, the more *effective* you are." What is God up to in this season of your life? What is He showing you that is being conceived in your life right now?

10 Tevet (DEC-JAN)

11 Sh'vat (JAN-FEB)

12 Adar (FEB-MAR)

WIN FOR THE MONTH

10 Tevet (DEC-JAN)

WEEK NO. 1:

WEEK NO. 2:

WEEK NO. 3:

WEEK NO. 4:

WIN FOR THE MONTH

11 Sh'vat (JAN-FEB)

WEEK NO. 1:

WEEK NO. 2:

WEEK NO. 3:

WEEK NO. 4:

WIN FOR THE MONTH

12 Adar (FEB-MAR)

WEEK NO. 1:

WEEK NO. 2:

WEEK NO. 3:

WEEK NO. 4:

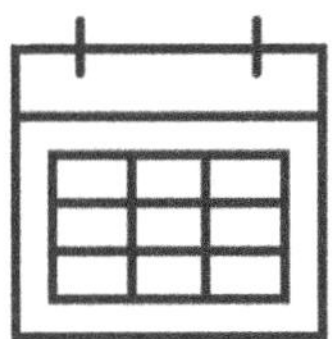

WINS FOR THE YEAR

THE ESSENTIALS

SPRING

Despite the rains often associated with Spring, it is a beautiful season, full of color and life. It is when things begin to bloom and flourish. Hope abounds. Spring signifies what is new, growing, or thriving in your life. It could be a new job, a new business venture, a new relationship, or a renewed relationship. These things bring joy and hope while simultaneously challenging, motivating, and astonishing you...even as they offer reasons to keep going.

1 Nissan (MAR-APR)

2 Iyyar (APR-MAY)

3 Sivan (MAY-JUN)

WIN FOR THE MONTH

1 Nissan (MAR-APR)

WEEK NO. 1:

WEEK NO. 2:

WEEK NO. 3:

WEEK NO. 4:

WIN FOR THE MONTH

2 Iyyar (APR-MAY)

WEEK NO. 1:

WEEK NO. 2:

WEEK NO. 3:

WEEK NO. 4:

WIN FOR THE MONTH

3 Sivan (MAY-JUN)

WEEK NO. 1:

WEEK NO. 2:

WEEK NO. 3:

WEEK NO. 4:

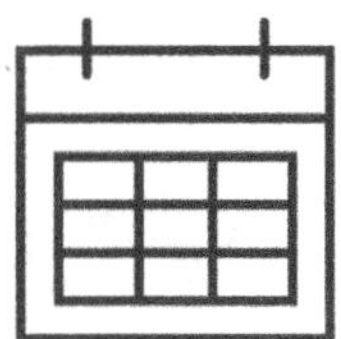

WINS FOR THE YEAR

THE ESSENTIALS

SUMMER

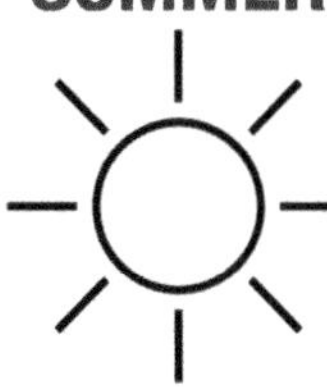

Summer is a season of sunshine and energy. It is also the time between sowing and reaping. Whatever "seeds" were sown in the Spring of your life requires two things during Summer: (1) pulling weeds and (2) watering seeds. "Weeds" are anything that prevents you from walking in alignment with God...and they must be removed at the root. Additionally, since nothing grows without water, whatever you planted in the Spring needs to be watered. What needs to be watered in your life?

4 Tammuz (JUN-JUL)

5 Av (JUL-AUG)

6 Elul (AUG-SEP)

WIN FOR THE MONTH

4 Tammuz (JUN-JUL)

WEEK NO. 1:

WEEK NO. 2:

WEEK NO. 3:

WEEK NO. 4:

WIN FOR THE MONTH

5 Av (JUL-AUG)

WEEK NO. 1:

WEEK NO. 2:

WEEK NO. 3:

WEEK NO. 4:

WIN FOR THE MONTH

6 Elul (AUG-SEP)

WEEK NO. 1:

WEEK NO. 2:

WEEK NO. 3:

WEEK NO. 4:

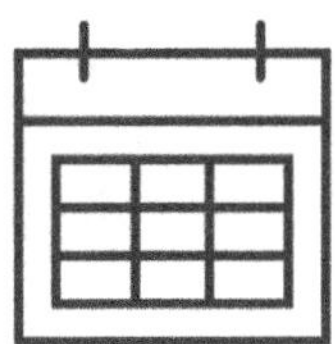

WINS FOR THE YEAR

THE ESSENTIALS

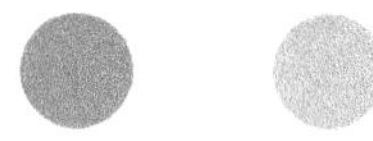

AUTUMN

The season of Autumn is a time to reap what was sown. Some of what we harvest is expected...and some is unexpected. It is a season to *rejoice* in what went well and *learn* from what did not end so well. We also need to avoid attempting to revive, through "weeding" and "watering", anything that has already died (e.g., remaining in toxic relationships, unsatisfying jobs, etc.). Instead, Autumn is the season to release those things and move forward.

7 Tishrei (SEP-OCT)

8 Cheshvan (OCT-NOV)

9 Kislev (NOV-DEC)

WIN FOR THE MONTH

7 Tishrei (SEP-OCT)

WEEK NO. 1:

WEEK NO. 2:

WEEK NO. 3:

WEEK NO. 4:

WIN FOR THE MONTH

8 Cheshvan (OCT-NOV)

WEEK NO. 1:

WEEK NO. 2:

WEEK NO. 3:

WEEK NO. 4:

WIN FOR THE MONTH

9 Kislev (NOV-DEC)

WEEK NO. 1:

WEEK NO. 2:

WEEK NO. 3:

WEEK NO. 4:

THE MINDSET TO THRIVE

Part 2

THE MINDSET TO THRIVE

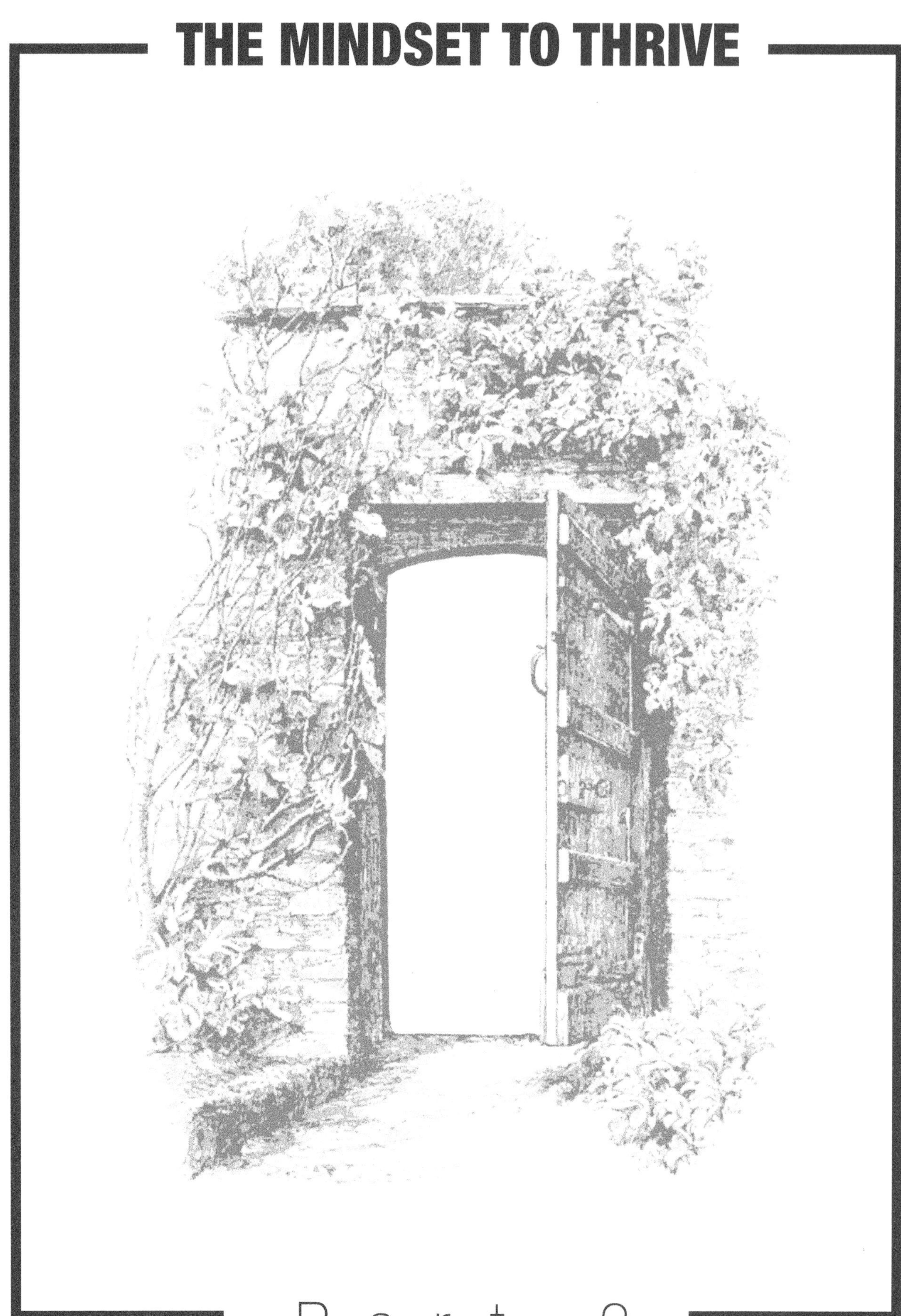

Part 2

CHOOSING YOUR MINDSET

A mindset is a habitual mental attitude that determines how we interpret and respond to life. Every time we choose to put our trust in God, we are building a mindset that prepares us to experience Him in a more intimate way. And over time, our minds and hearts become increasingly united with His.

> **DEUTERONOMY 11:18 CJB** | [18] Therefore, you are to store up these words of mine *in your heart* and *in all your being*;

> **HEBREWS 3:1 CJB** | [1] Therefore, brothers whom God has set apart, who share in the call from heaven, *think carefully* about Yeshua [Jesus], whom we acknowledge publicly as God's emissary and as cohen gadol [high priest].

It should come as no surprise then, that the battle for our minds (or mindsets) is the most important arena of spiritual warfare. This is why God says...

> **PROVERBS 3:5 CJB** | [5] Trust in ADONAI with *all your heart*; do not rely on your own understanding.

> **PROVERBS 4:23 CJB** | [23] Above everything else, *guard your heart*; for it is the source of life's consequences.

But protecting ourselves against the mindset of the world and devoting our heart to God requires trust. So, *where is our trust*? In God...or somewhere else?

How we respond to the world around us is directed by both the conscious and unconscious functions of the mindset that drives our thoughts and actions. Consequently, healing and growth in every aspect of our lives is *determined by the degree to which our minds have been transformed by God*.

> **ROMANS 12:2 CJB** | [2] In other words, do not let yourselves be conformed to the standards of the 'olam hazeh [Greek age]. Instead, keep letting yourselves be *transformed by the renewing of your minds*; so that you will know what God wants and will agree that what he wants is good, satisfying, and able to succeed.

Generally, there are three mindsets: (1) Barbarian, (2) Greek, or (3) Hebrew.

CHOOSING YOUR MINDSET

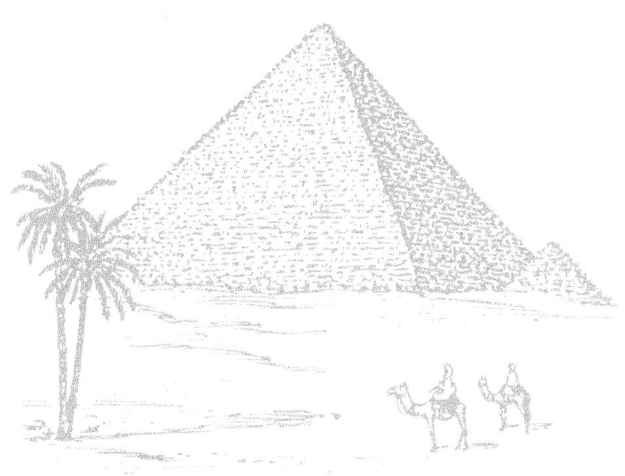

The world of the Old Testament was largely ruled by a **Barbarian Mindset** whose basic operating principle was FEAR...*because fearful people are easily manipulated and controlled.*

This is arguably the Adversary's favorite tactic because he is an oppressor by nature who loves to steal, kill, and enslave. He holds humanity (and even some believers) in such fear that they are unable (or unwilling) to resist him. [Why do so many of God's people resist learning intercessory prayer and avoid engagement in spiritual warfare?]

The **Barbarian Mindset** is perhaps most clearly illustrated by the pagan kings of the ancient Middle East who ruthlessly governed as tyrants and exerted absolute control over their terrified subjects. Modern terrorism was birthed from such a mindset, because fearful "sheeple" are easily dominated.

Whenever we make an agreement with fear, we are subjecting ourselves to the enemy's control. BUT if we resist him, the enemy flees. The good news: *The power of a lie lasts only as long as it is believed.*

However, since it is impossible to walk in both fear and faith at the same time, we must be intentional about choosing faith.

> **ROMANS 8:15 CJB** | [15] For you did not receive a spirit of slavery to bring you back again into fear; on the contrary, you received the Spirit, who makes us sons and by whose power we cry out, "Abba!" (that is, "Dear Father!").

> **2 TIMOTHY 1:7 CJB** | [7] For God gave us a Spirit who produces not timidity, but power, love, and self-discipline.

> **1 JOHN 4:18 CJB** | [18] There is no fear in love. On the contrary, love that has achieved its goal gets rid of fear, because fear has to do with punishment; the person who keeps fearing has not been brought to maturity in regard to love.

CHOOSING YOUR MINDSET

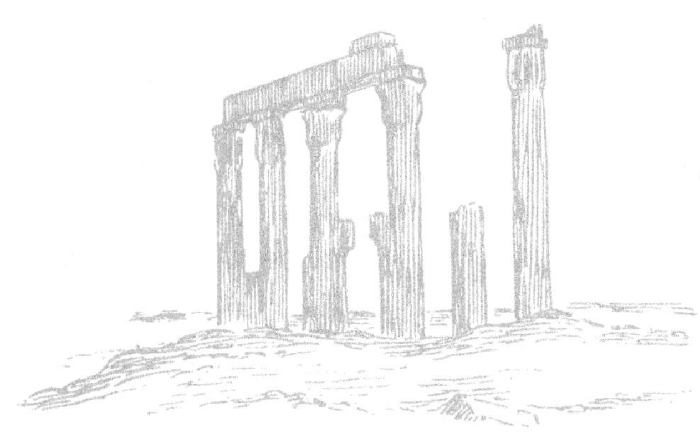

The world of the New Testament was largely ruled by a **Greek Mindset**. The polytheism practiced by the Greeks worshipped multiple gods created in the image of man. This mindset said, "We're our own gods who possess the power within ourselves to create a perfect world in which everyone works together toward the highest good."

PRIDE is the operating principle of this mindset, and it filters everything through a humanistic perspective. Consequently, the Greeks believed that knowledge was power. Therefore, IF a thing could be understood, THEN the outcome could be controlled and manipulated.

A **Greek Mindset** also reduced the intellect to "in-the-box" and "by-the-book" thinking. This is the Adversary's "Plan B." Although preferring the fear tactics of oppression, he will happily exploit a **Greek Mindset** to convince someone that "they're doing good"...while preventing them from experiencing God's best. In this way, "good" becomes the enemy of great.

Moreover, a **Greek Mindset** worships human reason and rejects anything that is "unscientifically explainable." Sadly, this mindset has become increasingly popular in the modern church, with the Holy Spirit, spiritual gifts, and miracles largely marginalized or simply ignored. As a result, many "believers" are living as practical agnostics who are misaligned with God's story for their lives.

> **ROMANS 1:21-22 CJB** | 21 "[...] On the contrary, they have become futile in their
> thinking; and their undiscerning hearts have become darkened. 22 Claiming to
> be wise, they have become fools!"

God *always* fulfills His promises but is not obligated to fulfill our potential. When He gives us a word...we must be willing to trust Him enough to follow where it leads. Although some lessons can *only* be learned in battle...God *only* invites us into battles that He's prepared us to win. Our victories strengthen our trust in Him and empower us to enter and remain in our "promised land."

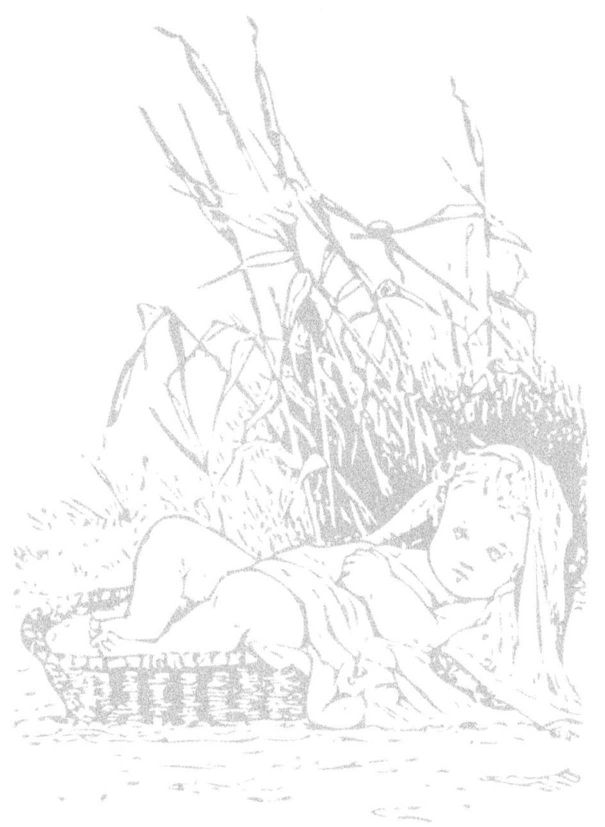

The **Hebrew Mindset** is a biblical mindset (and does not require you to be Jewish). It is the state of one whose thinking has been transformed by God's truth. For thousands of years, He shaped the Jewish culture to bring them into deeper alignment with His heart and mindset. And God is calling us into the same journey.

ISAIAH 55:8, 11 CJB | 8 "For my thoughts are not your thoughts, and your ways are not my ways," says ADONAI. [...] 11 so is my word that goes out from my mouth — it will not return to me unfulfilled; but it will accomplish what I intend, and cause to succeed what I sent it to do."

God instilled a biblical cycle of life into the Hebrew heart by celebrating the Sabbath, *Rosh-Chodesh*, and the high festivals...weekly, monthly, and yearly.

God gifted the nation of Israel with practical wisdom for success and showed them how to prosper in order to demonstrate to the world the blessing of being His people. In this way, God taught them a new mindset and established a new way of life that no other nation had ever seen before.

The operating principle of the **Hebrew Mindset** is trust in God. Through this trust, we are rewarded with the priceless gift of having our heart, mind, soul, and spirit united with His. And the more deeply we experience God's love, the more we are transformed into alignment with His purposes. However, both the **Barbarian** and **Greek Mindsets** view this transformation as foolishness.

1 CORINTHIANS 1:18 CJB | 18 For the message about the execution-stake is nonsense to those in the process of being destroyed, but to us in the process of being saved it is the power of God.

How Did Western Christianity Lose The Hebrew Mindset?

> It is important that we know where we come from, because if you do not know where you come from, then you don't know where you are, and if you don't know where you are, you don't know where you're going. And if you don't know where you're going, you're probably going wrong.
> TERRY PRATCHETT

The point that Mr. Pratchett is making here is rather profound and we will consider his observation in the context of questions like, "how did this happen and why does it matter?" "When (and how) did we forget?" and "At what cost? To our faith? To our families?"

According to Scripture, the Hebraic roots of Christianity extend all the way back to God's original covenant with Abram (c. 1800 BC)...[ALL EMPHASIS MINE].

> **GENESIS 12:2-3 CJB** | 2 "I [God] will make of you [Abram] a great nation, I will bless you, and I will make your name great; and you are to be a blessing. 3 I will bless those who bless you, but I will curse anyone who curses you; and by you ALL THE FAMILIES of the earth will be blessed."

A covenant that God later expanded upon...

> **GENESIS 17:1-7 CJB** | 1 [...] ADONAI appeared to Avram [Abram] and said to him, "I am El Shaddai [God Almighty]. Walk in my presence and be pure-hearted. 2 I will make my covenant between me and you, and I will increase your numbers greatly." 3 Avram fell on his face, and God continued speaking with him:
>
> 4 "As for me, this is my covenant with you: you will be the FATHER OF MANY NATIONS. 5 Your name will no longer be Avram [exalted father], but your name will be Avraham [Abraham, father of many], because I have made you the FATHER OF MANY NATIONS. 6 I will cause you to be very fruitful. I will make NATIONS OF YOU; kings will descend from you.

[7] "I am establishing my covenant between me and you, along with YOUR DESCENDANTS after you, generation after generation, as an EVERLASTING COVENANT, to be God for you and for YOUR DESCENDANTS after you."

Isaiah's prophesy (c. 1300 BC) confirmed that the fulfillment of God's covenant with Abraham would come through Jesus...

ISAIAH 11:1 CJB | [11] But a branch will emerge from the trunk of Yishai [Jesse], a shoot will grow from his roots.

And it was in Jesus that both Jew and Gentile were fully grafted.

ROMANS 11:17-18 CJB | [17] But if some of the branches were broken off, and you [Gentiles]—a wild olive—were grafted in among them [Jews] and have become equal sharers in the rich root [Yeshua] of the olive tree, [18] then don't boast as if you were better than the branches! However, if you do boast, remember that you are not supporting the root, the ROOT is supporting you.

Being grafted into Jesus (the root) represented the fulfillment of God's covenant with Abraham that brought Jew and Gentile together into His inheritance...

EPHESIANS 3:6 CJB | [6] that in UNION with the Messiah and through the Good News the Gentiles were to be JOINT HEIRS, a JOINT BODY and JOINT SHARERS with the Jews in what God has promised.

Moreover, Jesus' sacrifice also satisfied the *Torah* [Law] for all time in order to fulfill the covenant that God had made with Abraham generations before.

GALATIANS 3:21-25 CJB | [21] Does this mean that the legal part of the Torah [Law] stands in opposition to God's promises? Heaven forbid! For if the legal part of the Torah which God gave had in itself the power to give life, then righteousness really would have come by legalistically following such a Torah. 22 But instead, the Tanakh ['Teaching' + 'Prophets' + 'Writings']— shuts up everything under sin; so that what had been promised might be given, on the basis of Yeshua [Jesus] the Messiah's trusting faithfulness, to those who continue to be trustingly faithful.

23 Now before the time for this trusting faithfulness came, we were imprisoned in subjection to the system which results from perverting the Torah into legalism, kept under guard until this yet-to-come trusting faithfulness would be revealed. 24 *Accordingly, the Torah functioned as a custodian until the Messiah came, so that we might be declared righteous on the ground of trusting and being faithful.* 25 *But now that the time for this trusting faithfulness has come, we are no longer under a custodian.*

Through Jesus, Jew and Gentile are completely unified into one body...

EPHESIANS 2:11-16 CJB | 11 Therefore, remember your former state: you Gentiles by birth — called the Uncircumcised by those who, merely because of an operation on their flesh, are called the Circumcised — 12 at that time had no Messiah. You were estranged from the national life of Isra'el. You were foreigners to the covenants embodying God's promise. You were in this world without hope and without God.

13 But now, you who were once far off have been brought near through the shedding of the Messiah's blood. 14 For he himself is our shalom [peace]— he has made us both ONE and has broken down the m'chitzah [the middle wall of the boundary fence] which divided us 15 by destroying in his own body the enmity occasioned by the Torah [Law], with its commands set forth in the form of ordinances. He did this in order to create in UNION WITH HIMSELF FROM THE TWO GROUPS A SINGLE NEW HUMANITY and thus make shalom [peace], 16 and in order to reconcile to God both in a SINGLE BODY by being executed on a stake as a criminal and thus in himself killing that enmity.

1 CORINTHIANS 12:12-13 CJB | 12 For just as the body is one but has many parts; and all the parts of the body, though many, constitute one body; so, it is with the Messiah. 13 For it was by one Spirit that we were all immersed into one

> body, WHETHER JEWS OR GENTILES, slaves or free; and we were ALL given the one Spirit to drink.

The Hebrew roots of the Christian faith are as certain as any Ancestry.com® DNA result.

Rediscovering the richness of both our identity and our inheritance enables us to more fully experience the presence of God in ever-increasing measure as we realign our hearts, minds, and spirits with Him.

Several years ago, when I [Daniel] attended The Master's University (a private Christian college), one of the required courses was "Christian Theology." On the first day of class, my professor posed a rather thought-provoking question, "How many of you know that *Christianity does not exist*?"

We were shocked by his seemingly blasphemous suggestion and immediately started peddling around on our religious Huffy® bikes. Fortunately, before we suffocated on our own self-righteousness, he continued:

"Jesus was born, lived, and died as a practicing Jew. Paul, who wrote most of the New Testament, was born, lived, and died as a practicing Jew. Likewise, the twelve Apostles who followed Jesus were born, lived and died as practicing Jews. At no point did Jesus, Paul, or the Twelve, ever attempt to establish a 'religion' called 'Christianity.'" He went on...

"However, Paul did go to great lengths, often at the risk of his life, to demonstrate that Jesus was the promised Messiah who had *fulfilled* the Law and who offered redemption to *both* Jew and Gentile. He wasn't founding 'Christianity'...he was attempting to reform Judaism."

The whole class was stunned. It made perfect sense, but why was this the first time we had ever heard such a thing? And why did Christianity forget its Hebrew roots? We'll need to go back nearly 1,900 years ago for the answer.

A compelling argument can be made that early Western Christianity widely embraced the belief that (1) Israel had been rejected by her God and (2) the

"Church" was now the new Israel.[1] This argument principally relied upon two major events that appeared to confirm this view:

- The destruction of the Jewish Temple in 70 AD under the direction of the **Roman Emperor Titus (39-81 AD)**.
- The destruction of the Jewish nation in 135 AD led by the false Messiah, Simon bar Kochba.

Following their defeat in the **Bar Kokhba Revolt (c. 132-136 AD)**, hundreds of thousands of Jews were massacred and most of the remaining survivors were dispersed into the *Gamut* ["Diaspora" or "Exile"]. Among those who managed to survive, many were sold into slavery. These events marked the beginning of the decline of Jewish influence on Western Christianity.

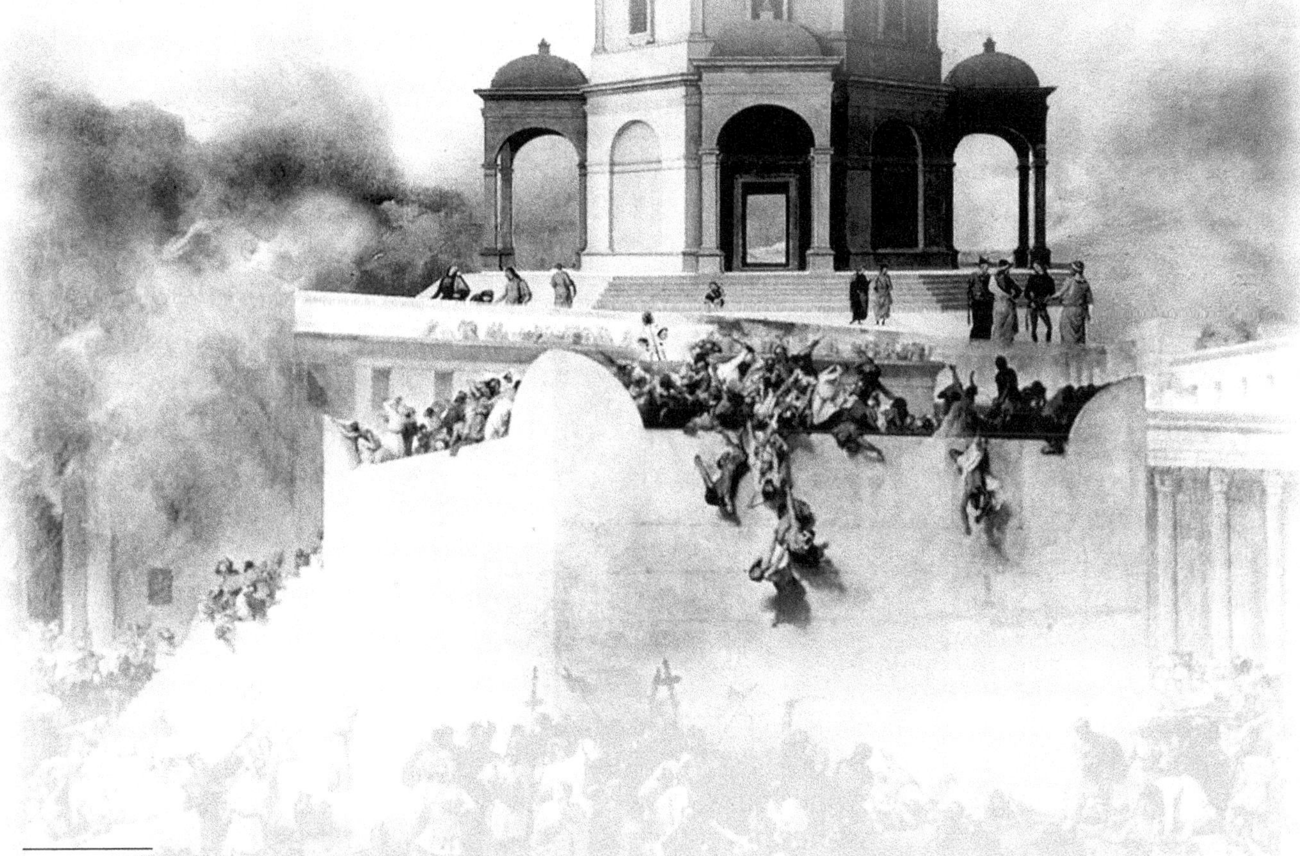

[1] This view evolved into modern "replacement theology" or "supersessionism, or "fulfillment theology"...a Protestant doctrine that asserts (1) Christianity succeeded the Israelites as "God's people" and (2) the New Covenant replaced or superseded the Mosaic covenant.

The Early Church Fathers Laid The Foundation For Anti-Semitism

[NOTE: *All italics are mine*]

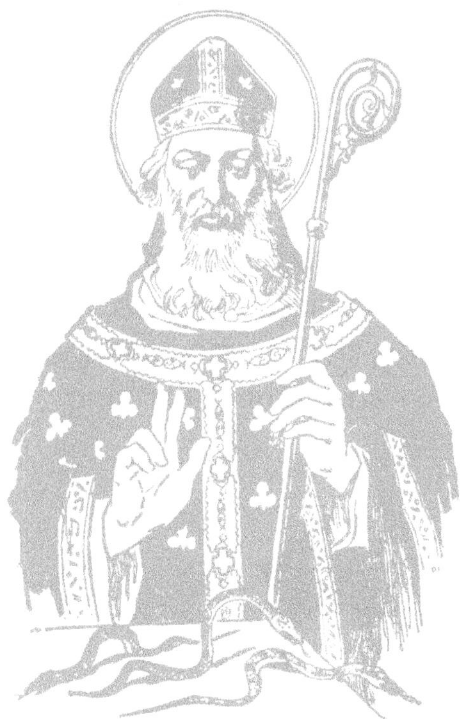

Bishop Ignatius of Antioch (c. 35-108 AD). In a letter to the Magnesians (modern-day Turkey), he said:

"To profess Jesus Christ while continuing to follow Jewish customs is an absurdity. The Christian faith does not look to Judaism, *Judaism looks to Christianity*, in which every other race and tongue that confesses a belief in God has not been comprehended."[2]

Justin Martyr (c. 100-165 AD). He claimed the Scriptures were "*not yours [the Jews], but ours [the Christians].*"[3]

Irenaeus (c. 130-202 AD). He wrote:

"[The Jews] indeed had they been cognizant of [Christians'] future existence, and that we should use these proofs from the Scriptures, would themselves never have hesitated to burn their own Scriptures, which do declare that all other nations partake of [eternal] life, and show that they who boast themselves as being the house of Jacob and the people of Israel, *are disinherited from the grace of God.*"[4]

---

[2] Maxwell Stamforth, trans., ed. Andrew Louth, *Early Christian Writings: The Apostolic Fathers* (New York, NY: Penguin Classics, 1968), p. 73.

[3] Justin Martyr, *Dialogue with Trypho*, trans. Marcus Dods & George Reith, rev. and ed. Kevin Knight, ch. 29, *New Advent*, www.newadvent.org/fathers/01282.htm (accessed 8 July 2018).

[4] *St. Irenaeus, Against Heresies*, trans. Alexander Roberts & William Rambaut, ed. Alexander Roberts, James Donaldson & A. Cleveland Coxe, rev. and ed. Kevin Knight, book 3, ch. 22, *New Advent*, www.newadvent.org/fathers/0103321.htm (accessed 8 July 2018).

Tertullian (c. 160-220 AD). He is credited with writing, "*God has rejected the Jews in favor of the Christians*"[5] and referred to the "synagogues of the Jews" as "fountains of persecution."

Origen of Alexandria (c. 184-253 AD). He wrote:

"We say with confidence that [the Jews] *will never be restored to their former condition*. For they committed a crime of the most unhallowed kind, in conspiring against the Savior of the human race. [...] It accordingly behooved that city where Jesus underwent these sufferings to perish utterly, and *the Jewish nation to be overthrown*, and the invitation to happiness offered them by God *to pass to others—the Christians, I mean.*"[6]

Eusebius of Caesarea (c. 263-339 AD). He wrote that, "The promises of the Hebrew Scriptures are *now for the Christians and not the Jews—but the curses are for the Jews.*"[7]

Augustine of Hippo (354-430 AD). He was one of the few early church fathers to offer support for the Jews, writing in *City of God* that they at least deserved respect and protection:

"By the evidence of their own scriptures they bear witness for us that we have not fabricated the prophecies about Christ. [...] It follows that when the Jews do not believe in our scriptures, their scriptures are fulfilled in them, while they read them with blind eyes. [...] It is in order to give this testimony which, in spite of themselves, they supply for our benefit by their possession and preservation of those books [the *Tanakh*] that they are themselves dispersed among all nations, wherever the Christian church spreads. [...]

---

[5] Earl Cox, "The True Face of Christendom," *Jerusalem Post* (7 February 2017), citing Tertullian's, "Against the Jews," www.jpost.com/Blogs/Israel-Uncensored/The-True-Face-of-Christendom-480779.

[6] Origen of Alexandria, *Contra Celsum*, trans. Frederick Crombie, rev. and ed. Kevin Knight, book 4, ch. 22, *New Advent*, www.newadvent.org/fathers/0416.htm (accessed 8 July 2018).

[7] Earl Cox, "The True Face of Christendom."

"Hence the prophecy in the *Book of Psalms*: 'Slay them not, lest they forget your law, scatter them by your might.'"[8]

But even Augustine's considerable influence was unable to prevent the seeds of anti-Semitism from blossoming into religious and political persecution.[9] In fact, by the time **Constantine (272-337 AD)** convened the first general church council at Nicaea in 325 AD, anti-Semitism had already become well-entrenched in the "Church." Is it by mere coincidence that none of the 318 bishops who attended the Nicaean Council were of Jewish ancestry?

Moreover, the anti-Judaic theology of Nicaea served to "legitimize" the anti-Semitic legislation of later church councils. For example:

- The **Council of Antioch (341 AD)** prohibited Christians from celebrating Passover with the Jews.

- The **Council of Laodicea (364 AD)** prohibited Christians from observing the Jewish (and biblical) Sabbath. (Some Christians had been observing both Sunday and the Sabbath.) It also prohibited Christians from receiving gifts from Jews or *matzah* [unleavened bread] from Jewish festivals and "impieties."[10]

Despite these restrictions, Judaism was not initially treated as a "prohibited sect"[11] and rabbis were granted the same privileges as Christian clergy. These laws also prevented Jews from being disturbed on their Sabbath or Feast Days, and protected their synagogues from being attacked, violated, burned, or confiscated. However, Jewish tribunals were considered valid only in religious matters and conversion was entirely a one-way street to Christianity.

---

[8] Augustine, *City of God*, 18.26; cf. Paula Fredricksen, *Augustine and the Jews: A Christian Defense of Jews and Judaism* (New Haven, CT: Yale University Press, 2010), xii.

[9] James Everett Seaver, *Persecution of the Jews in the Roman Empire* (Lawrence, KS: University of Kansas Publications, 1952).

[10] Michael W. Holmes, trans., *Apostolic Fathers in English* (Grand Rapids, MI: Baker Academic, 2006), p. 357.

[11] Cf. *Codex Theodosianus* (438 AD).

- Jews were encouraged to convert to Christianity, BUT Christians were forbidden to convert to Judaism.
- Christians were permitted to own Jewish slaves, BUT Jews were forbidden from owning Christian slaves.
- Christians were forbidden under penalty of death to marry Jews.
- The *Fiscus Judaicus*[12] [Jewish tax] was reinstituted from earlier centuries.

The limited protections offered by the *Codex Judaicus* would be relatively short-lived. Within a few decades, violence against Jews and their synagogues was commonplace and they were reduced to little more than second-class citizens (somewhat protected by law and only barely tolerated).

Constantine "Saves" Christianity

Although Constantine technically "converted" to Christianity, he remained a devout Mithraist (i.e., worshipper of Mithra, the 'sun-god') to the end of his life.[13]

It should be noted that the triumphal arch he built in Rome (c. 315 AD) was adorned with the symbols of the "Unconquered Sun"...NOT Christianity.

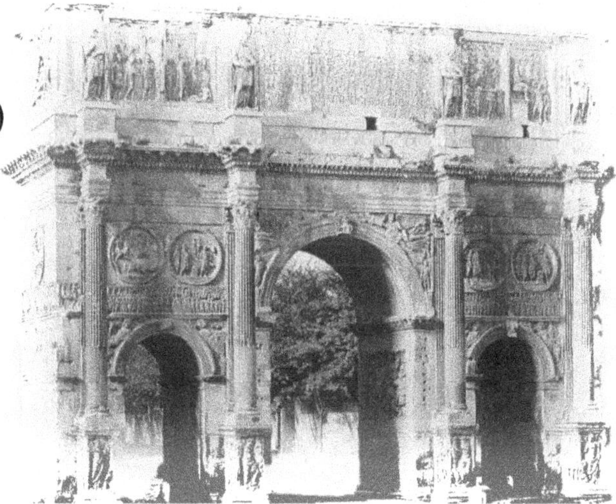

Constantine also placed sculptures of river gods and depictions of the Sun (east) above the two small arches.

---

[12] A tax-collection agency instituted to collect taxes imposed on Jews in the Roman Empire following the destruction of Jerusalem and its Temple in 70 AD. After the revenues had been collected, they were directed to the Temple of Jupiter Optimus Maximus in Rome.

[13] ENCYCLOPEDIA BRITANNICA | The worship of Mithra, Iranian god of the sun, justice, contract, and war in pre-Zoroastrian Iran was known as Mithras in the Roman Empire during the 2nd and 3rd centuries AD. This deity was honoured as the patron of loyalty to the emperor.

Although the "Christian" emperor did indeed reform several aspects of pagan cult worship, he continued to promote their traditions and practices. For example, in 321 AD he declared the "Day of the Sun" to be a state holiday celebrated by Roman citizens.

Moreover, Constantine's reign was far more political than spiritual in nature and largely concerned itself with forging alliances between church and state to maintain social stability throughout the empire.

In 313 AD, Constantine met with Licinius in Italy to formulate the **Edict of Milan**, which legalized Christianity...along with *all other religions and cults in the Roman Empire*. However, once Christianity was granted this official recognition, Christians were no longer targeted for persecution by the pagans.[14]

In 325 AD, the **Nicene Council**[15] was convened to create a universal religion/church in order to strengthen the Roman empire. As emperor, Constantine presided over the entire council whose representation was conspicuously greater among the wealthier churches, since the poorer ones could not afford the exorbitant expense of sending emissaries more than a thousand miles to attend.

> "Some bishops, blinded by the splendor of the court, even went so far as to laud the emperor as an angel of God, as a sacred being, and to prophesy that he would, like the Son of God, reign in heavens.[16]
>
> CATHOLIC ENCYCLOPEDIA

---

[14] Sadly, Christians used this new-found freedom to persecute others (including other Christians) with a relentless zeal. In fact, more Christians were killed (by other Christians!) in the first century after the Council of Nicaea than had been killed by pagans in the century preceding Nicaea.

[15] The 20 canons of Nicaea are quoted verbatim here, with brief editorial notes attached to each one. www.christian-history.org/council-of-nicea-canons.html.

[16] *Catholic Encyclopedia*, Vol. 4, "Constantine."

After Nicaea, the "Christian Emperor" quickly cast aside his "faith" in order to ruthlessly consolidate political power:[17]

- In 325 AD, Constantine had Licinius (the husband of his half-sister) strangled and the son of Licinius flogged to death.
- In 326 AD, Constantine had Crispus (his first-born son) strangled.
- Later that same year, Constantine had Fausta (his second wife) boiled alive.

The words of Hyam Maccoby are an especially apt description of Constantine's so-called faith, "*Nothing is more welcome to a military empire than a religious doctrine that counsels' obedience and acquiescence.*"[18]

Given his parricidal tendencies, it seems quite clear that Constantine retained a considerable measure of his pagan inclinations, since it was also during his reign that:

- The cross[19] became a sacred symbol in Christianity and some scholars have even suggested it was alternatively used in various pagan religions.[20]
- An edict declaring the "Venerable Day of the Sun" (Sunday) was issued at the Council of Nicaea.[21]

Although Passover continued to be celebrated by the Christian church, Gentiles began to differentiate "their Passover" from the Jewish Passover. To complete this transition, the bishops moved the Christian celebration of Passover to the first Sunday after the Jewish Passover (in most years).[22]

---

[17] Ralph Woodrow, *Babylon Mystery Religion* (Ralph Woodrow Association, 1981), pp. 55-59.

[18] Hyam Maccoby, *The Mythmaker: Paul and the invention of Christianity* (1998), p. 163.

[19] The Jews referred to this alternatively as a "tree" ['ets] or "execution stake."

[20] Ibid., pp. 47-54. Cf. William Wood Seymour, *The Cross in Tradition, History, and Art* (New York, NY: G. P. Putnam's Sons, 1897), pp. 9-26.

[21] Until this time, both Jewish and Gentile Christians generally observed the seventh day Sabbath (cf. EXODUS 20:8-11; LEVITICUS 23:3; DEUTERONOMY 5:12-14; EZEKIEL 20:19-20; ISAIAH 58:13-1).

[22] The Jewish Passover always lands on the 14th day of Abib (Nissan), which can fall on any day of the week.

Centuries later, even the name of *Pesach* [Passover] became so distasteful to the Christian church that they replaced it with Easter (the name of a pagan fertility goddess).[23]

By this time, the practice of "Christening" was already widely believed to make one a "Christian" and by 416 AD, infant baptism had become compulsory for the entire Roman Empire. Any followers of Jesus who rejected this law were forbidden from identifying as Christian because they had not been "christened" into Christendom. Those guilty of committing this "heresy" were often punished by death.

In truth, Western Christianity was really no different than any other historical group, religious or otherwise: there was blood on its hands. While the excesses of the Roman Catholic Church are rightfully condemned, neither should the uglier aspects of historical Protestantism be conveniently ignored. We are *all* human, are we not? Consequently, it behooves us to avoid the arrogant indulgence of believing that theological errors and religious excesses are exclusively confined to "other religions."

Why Is Greek, Not Hebrew, The Language Of The New Testament?

Biblical scholars generally believe that the 27 books comprising the New Testament were composed in *Koine* Greek.[24] But this form of Greek is better understood as Judeo-*Koine* Greek, a linguistic combination of sorts similar to that of Judeo-German (Yiddish), Judeo-Spanish (Ladino), etc. In other words, it was a form of Greek used by Jews to communicate.

Consequently, this dialectical form retained several words, phrases, grammatical structures, and thought patterns characteristic of the Hebrew

---

[23] In "De temporum ratione" ("The Reckoning of Time"), English monk Bede (672-735 AD), the "father of English history," wrote that pagans in England called April, "Ēosturmōnaþ" (Old English for the "Month of Ēostre"). This "Christian" holiday, now known as Easter, "was called after a goddess of theirs named Ēostre, in whose honor feasts were celebrated in that month." Ēostre was alternatively known as a goddess of fertility, dawn, or light.

[24] This is a different linguistic form of Classical Greek and was the common multi-regional form of Greek spoken and written during Hellenistic and Roman antiquity.

language. So, not only was the New Testament written with a Hebrew mindset, but the primary source for their Old Testament quotations were taken from another Jewish-authored document, the *Septuagint*.

In addition to the *Septuagint*, the oldest existing copies of the Masoretic Text (authoritative Hebrew/Aramaic text of the 24 books of *Tanakh* for Rabbinic Judaism) date back to the 10th century and two important pieces of textual evidence support its accuracy:

- The successive discoveries of scrolls at Qumran[26] revealed portions of manuscripts several centuries older than any previously known.
- The comparison of the Masoretic text to the Septuagint (c. 200-150 BC) confirmed its accuracy, with the oldest existing manuscripts dating back to the 4th century AD.

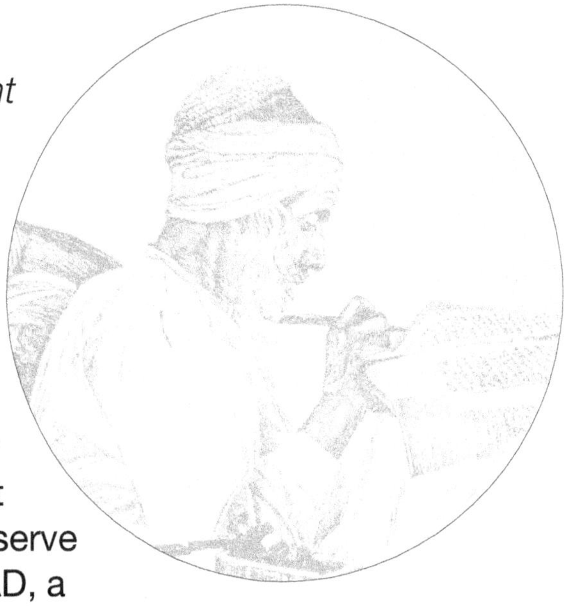

Both the Dead Sea Scrolls and the *Septuagint* revealed an amazing consistency with the Masoretic Text which offers reliable assurance that God divinely protected His Word through thousands of years of copying and translating.

Interestingly, the earliest copies of the Hebrew Bible were written without vowels or accents, as written Hebrew did not represent vowels until the Middle Ages. In order to preserve traditional spoken readings, starting c. 400 AD, a group of Jewish scribes known as the Masoretes carefully selected, copied, and annotated biblical scrolls, adding vowels and accents to the ancient Hebrew consonants in the process.

Although Masoretic scribes added these vowels to the original text long after it had been written, they were likely preserving traditional vocalizations (writing)

[26] A collection of ancient writings recorded by an Essene community that lived in the West Bank near the Dead Sea (c. 200-100 BC) and were first discovered in 1947.

in vowels) that dated to much earlier times and eventually produced several different systems of vocalization sometime between 500 and 700 AD.

The discovery of the Dead Sea Scrolls also suggested that there were different versions of several biblical books from the Second Temple period (530 BC to 70 AD). Some of these versions were nearly identical, while other versions were quite different.

Following the destruction of Jerusalem and its temple by the Romans in 70 AD, Jewish groups dispersed across the ancient world, preserving these versions of the Hebrew Scriptures in their communities. One of these groups preserved the texts that would later become the Masoretic Text. Others are preserved in versions such as the *Septuagint*, the earliest Greek translation.

In the 10th century AD, the ben Asher scribal family of Tiberias produced a manuscript of the Hebrew Bible that famed Jewish scholar **Maimonides (1138-1204)** declared to be the best-known version of the sacred text. Shortly thereafter, the Tiberian Masoretic text and its particular version of vowels and annotations became the standard, authoritative text of the Hebrew Bible for rabbinic Judaism.[27]

The Masoretic Text is the version held as authoritative and used liturgically in most synagogues today. The Catholic Church since the time of **Jerome (347-420 AD)** and most Protestant Christian churches also use this version as their source text for modern translations.

However, Professor Gershon Galil, of the Department of Biblical Studies at the University of Haifa deciphered an inscription that, "indicates that the Kingdom of Israel *already existed in the 10th century BC* and that at least some of the biblical texts were written *hundreds of years before the dates presented in current research*."

---

[27] The two most important Masoretic medieval manuscripts are the *Aleppo Codex* (c. 900 AD), and the *Leningrad Codex* (1009 AD).

This discovery is the earliest known Hebrew writing to date and its significance cannot be understated because it demonstrates that (1) at least some of the biblical scriptures were composed hundreds of years before scholars had previously thought and (2) the Kingdom of Israel was already in existence at that time.

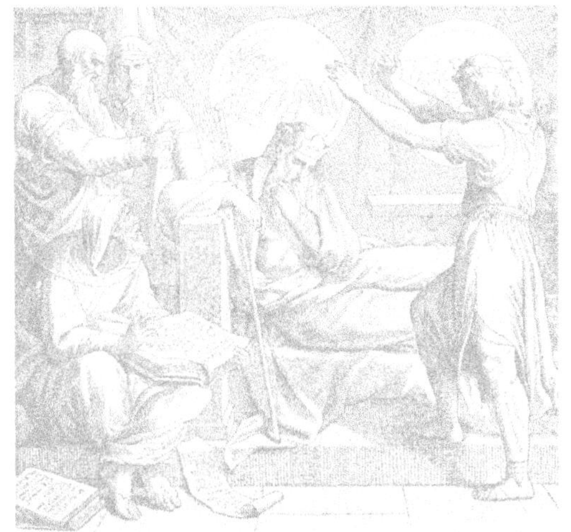

The inscription itself, excavated in 2008 by Professor Yosef Garfinkel at Khirbet Qeiyafa near the Valley of Elah, was written in ink on a 15cm x 16.5cm trapezoid pottery shard and dated back to the 10th century BC (during King David's reign).

Professor Galil's deciphering of the ancient writing testified to its being Hebrew, based on the use of verbs particular to the Hebrew language, and content specific to Hebrew culture and not adopted by any other cultures in the region.

> “This text is a social statement, relating to slaves, widows and orphans. It uses verbs that were characteristic of Hebrew, such as *asah* ('did') and *avad* ('worked'), which were rarely used in other regional languages. Particular words that appear in the text, such as *almanah* ('widow') are specific to Hebrew and are written differently in other local languages. The content itself was also unfamiliar to all the cultures in the region besides the Hebrew society: The present inscription provides social elements similar to those found in the biblical prophecies and very different from prophecies written by other cultures postulating glorification of the gods and taking care of their physical needs.[28]
>
> GERSHON GALIL

---

[28] Although clearly not copied from any biblical text, the content of the inscription is similar to content in ISAIAH 1:17, PSALMS 72:3, EXODUS 23:3, et. al.

He also noted that since the inscription was discovered in a provincial town in Judea, it could be reasoned that if scribes resided in the periphery, then those inhabiting the central region and Jerusalem were even more proficient writers.

> "It can now be maintained that it was highly reasonable that during the 10th century BC, during the reign of King David, there were scribes in Israel who were able to write literary texts and complex historiographies such as the books of Judges and Samuel.
>
> GERSHON GALIL

Given the complexity of the text discovered in Khirbet Qeiyafa, along with the impressive fortifications revealed at the site, it is almost certain that the Kingdom of Israel already existed at that time.

Additionally, a recent study[29] published by Tel Aviv University (TAU) doctoral students Shira Faigenbaum-Golovina, Arie Shausa, and Barak Sober (*Proceedings of the National Academy of Sciences*) suggests that the Hebrew Scriptures were likely written earlier than previously thought.

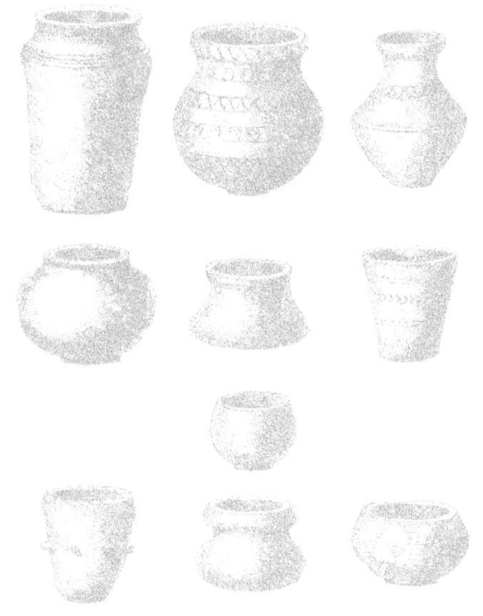

The TAU researchers analyzed multi-spectral images of sixteen Hebrew inscriptions, which were written in ink on ostraca (broken pottery pieces), using a computer software program they developed. The ostraca, which date to 600 BC, were excavated from the Judahite fortress at Tel Arad in southern Israel. [SIDE NOTE: This was one of the places our family prayed at when we visited Israel in 2018].

The researchers claim they were able to identify at least six different styles of handwriting on the inscriptions, which contained instructions for troop movements and lists of food expenses.

---

[29] Robin Ngo, "When Was the Hebrew Bible Written? Earlier than previously thought, say Tel Aviv University researchers," *Bible History Daily* (10 May 2017).

They also noted that, "the tone and nature of the commands precluded the role of professional scribes" the research team concluded, "The results indicate that in this remote fort, *literacy had spread throughout the military hierarchy*, down to the quartermaster and probably even below that rank."

According to TAU Professor of Archaeology Israel Finkelstein, who heads the research project, "Adding what we know about Arad to other forts and administrative localities across ancient Judah, we can estimate that *many people could read and write during the last phase of the First Temple period*. We assume that in a kingdom of some 100,000 people, at least several hundred were literate."

Curators at the Israel Museum have called "Gabriel's Revelation" the most important document since the Dead Sea Scrolls were discovered in 1947. While this may be an interesting sidebar into the field of biblical archaeology, *what does literacy in the Iron Age have to do with the Hebrew Scriptures*?

Scholars have long debated whether the Hebrew Scriptures were composed before 586 BC—when the Babylonians destroyed Jerusalem, razed the First Temple, and exiled the Jews—or later—during the Persian or Hellenistic periods. However, IF literacy in Iron Age Judah was more widespread than previously thought, this could mean that Hebrew scriptural texts were written BEFORE the Babylonian conquest.

The researchers at Tel Aviv University certainly think so, based on their examination of the ostraca from Arad.

However, their conclusions are not without detractors. Epigrapher Christopher Rollston, Associate Professor of Northwest Semitic languages and literatures at George Washington University, published a lengthy blog analysis of the TAU study in which he contends the ostraca contain insufficient information to accurately assess the literacy of Iron Age Judah.

Rollston adds that Yohanan Aharoni, the original excavator at Arad, determined that the sixteen ostraca came from different strata dated across the 7th and early 6th centuries—and therefore do not all date to 600 BC.

Although Rallston disagrees with the specific conclusions of the TAU researchers, he allows that there is enough epigraphic evidence from ancient Israel to conclude, "*already by 800 BC there was sufficient intellectual infrastructure*, that is, well-trained scribes, able to produce sophisticated historical and literary texts."[30]

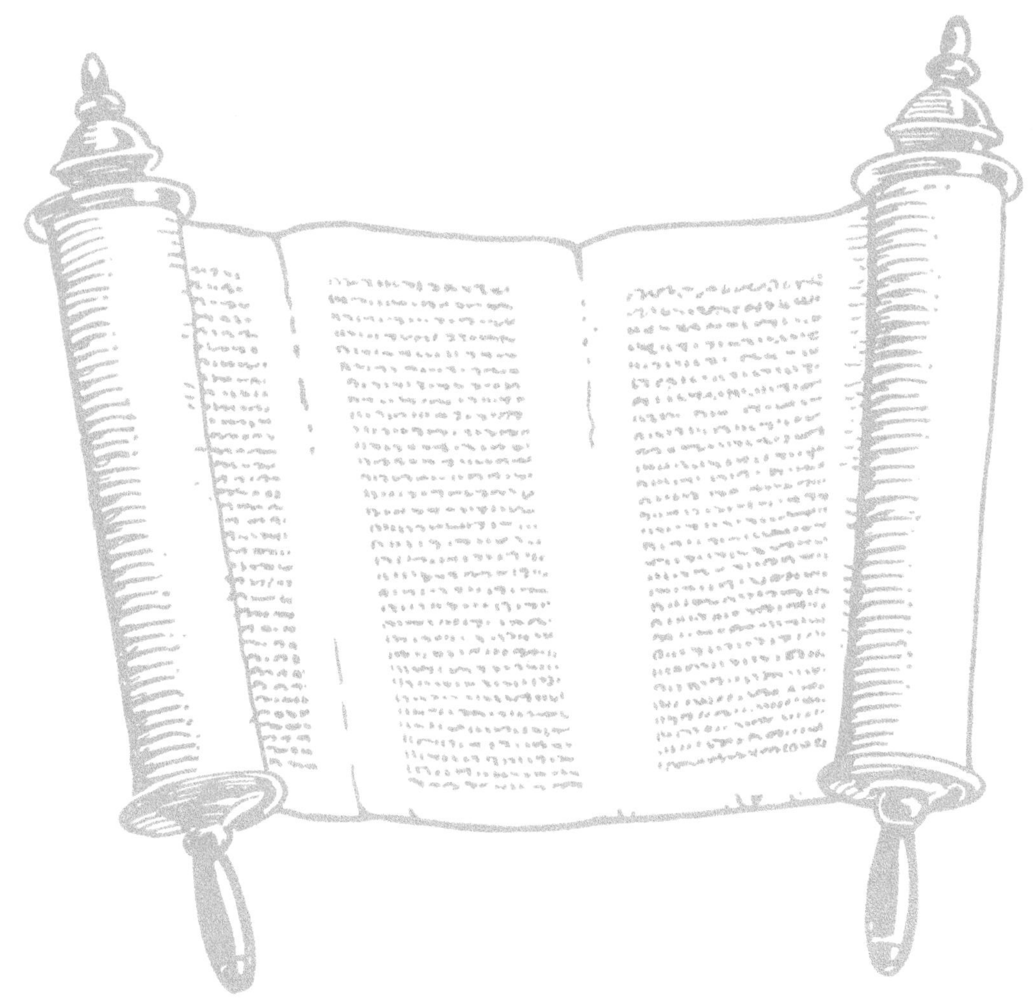

---

[30] Substantive scholarly arguments in favor of early dating for the Torah have also been made by William M. Schniedewind, *How the Bible Became a Book: The Textualization of Ancient Isra*el (Cambridge, UK; Cambridge University Press, 2003) and Seth L. Sanders, *The Invention of Hebrew (Traditions)* (Chicago, IL: University of Illinois Press, 2011).

THE RHYTHMS OF GOD

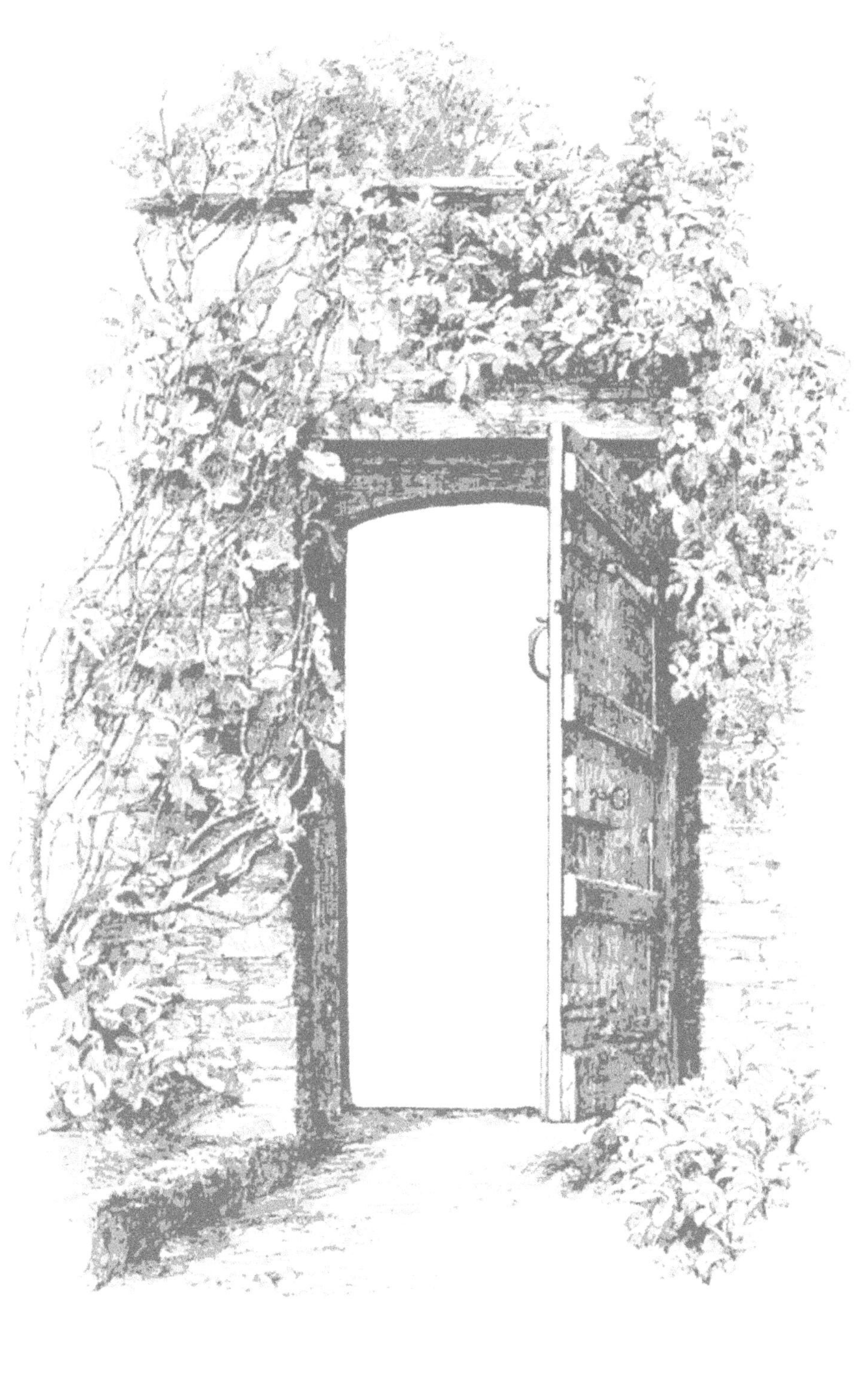

Part 3

THE RHYTHMS OF GOD

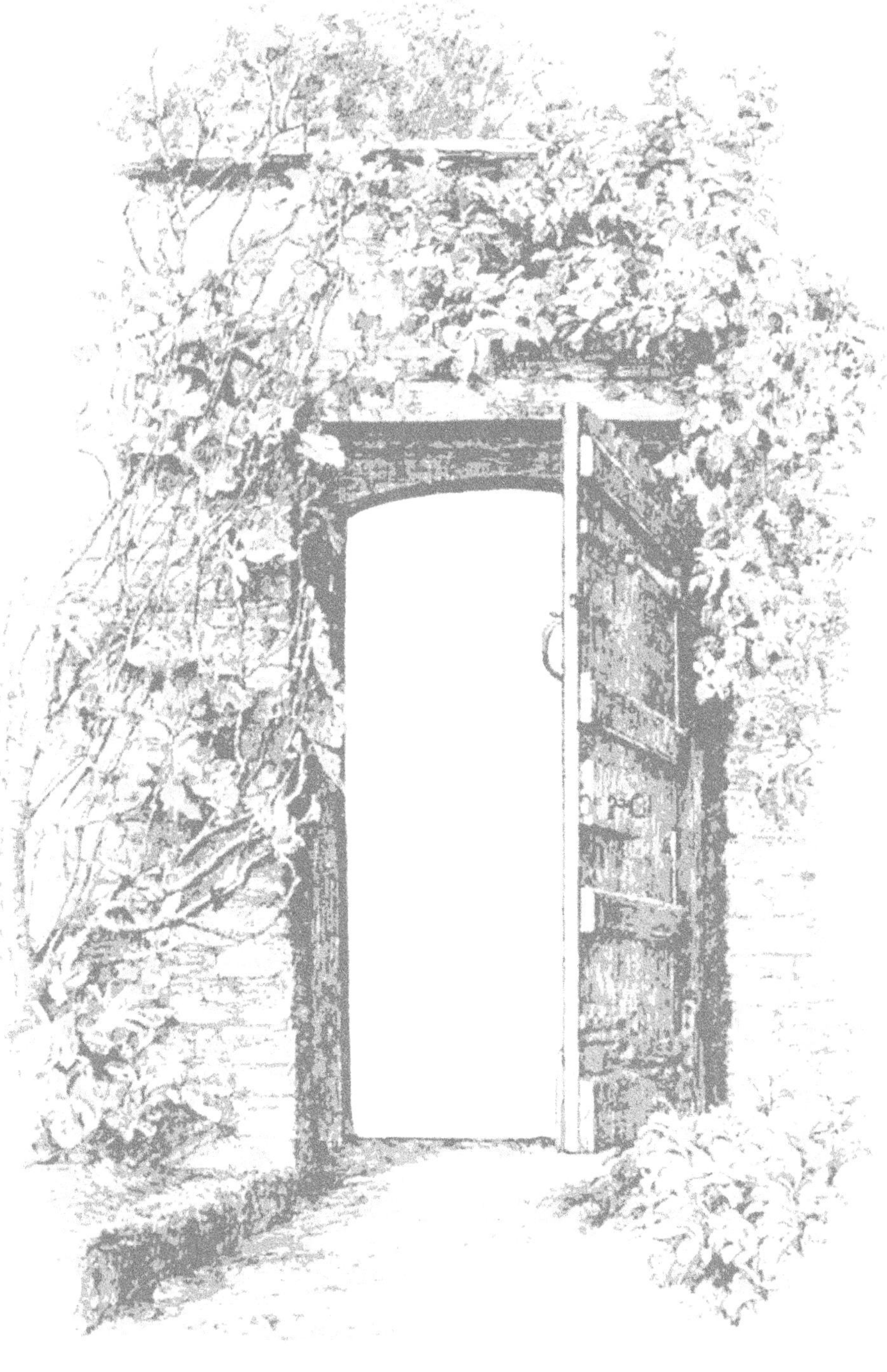

Part 3

According to Hebrew tradition, the twelve constellations illustrate God's sovereignty over creation and the cosmic order. Consequently, Jews viewed the constellations as reflections of His creative power to orchestrate the times and seasons and were NEVER intended as an instrument of occultic, astrological fortune-telling.

> **GENESIS 1:14-19 CJB** | 14 God said, "Let there be lights in the dome of the sky to divide the day from the night; let them be for signs, seasons, days and years; 15 and let them be for lights in the dome of the sky to give light to the earth"; and that is how it was.
>
> 16 God made the two great lights — the larger light to rule the day and the smaller light to rule the night — and the stars. 17 God put them in the dome of the sky to give light to the earth, 18 to rule over the day and over the night, and to divide the light from the darkness; and God saw that it was good.

In reality, the constellations point to God's divine truth, and each one is aligned with the twelve tribes, the twelve months, and key spiritual themes that recur throughout Israel's history.

This perspective underscores a worldview where God's supremacy over both the visible and invisible realms is absolute...a theme thoroughly explored by Old Testament scholars like Dr. Michael S. Heiser and Dr. G. K. Beale who view the zodiac constellations as signs of God's interaction with His creation rather than mystical guides to secret knowledge.

Interestingly, the Hebrew word "mazzaroth" [Strong's H4216] directly refers to the twelve signs of the zodiac and their 36 associated constellations, which include Ursa Major, Orion, and the Pleiades.

These constellations are mentioned twice in the book of Job...

> **JOB 9:9 CJB** | 9 He [God] made the Great Bear, Orion, the Pleiades and the hidden constellations of the south.

And then later, in God's interrogation of Job...

JOB 38:31-33 CJB | [31] "Can you [Job] tie up the cords of the Pleiades or loosen the belt of Orion? [32] Can you lead out the constellations of the zodiac [mazzaroth] in their season or guide the Great Bear and its cubs? [33] Do you know the laws of the sky? Can you determine how they affect the earth?

These references were familiar to the ancient Hebrews and reinforced their understanding of God's authority over the celestial bodies, with each constellation representing an aspect of His divine order and purpose. For instance, Ursa Major ["Great Bear"], is a constellation of the northern sky whose seven brightest stars constitute one of the most famous astronomical bodies...the Big Dipper.

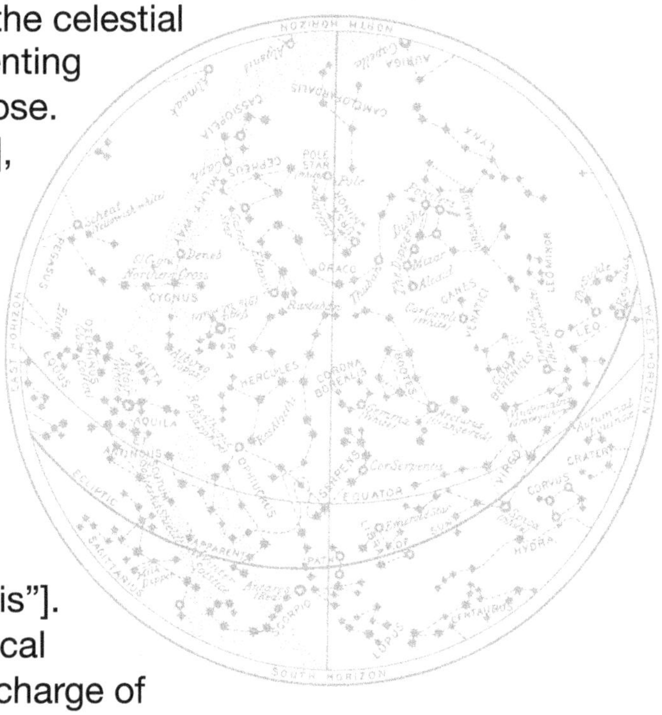

The constellation of Orion is one of the fifteen equatorial constellations and contains two of the ten brightest stars in the night sky, Rigel ["Beta Orionis"] and Betelgeuse ["Alpha Orionis"]. Orion is typically depicted in astronomical maps as a hunter who is (a) facing the charge of the bull (Taurus), (b) pursuing the Pleiades sisters (the famed open star cluster), or (c) chasing the hare ["Lepus"] with his two hunting dogs, represented in the nearby Canis Major and Canis Minor.

The Pleiades, an open cluster in the Taurus constellation, holds over 1,000 stars of which six (or sometimes seven) are visible to the naked eye. In the Northern Hemisphere, the heliacal (i.e., near dawn) rising of the Pleiades in spring marks the beginning of the seafaring and farming seasons, as the morning setting of the cluster in autumn signifies the seasons' end.

According to rabbinical scholars, these twelve constellations illustrate God's sovereign order in creation. Far from being used for occultic practices such as astrology, these constellations were designed to (1) reflect God's power over times and seasons and (2) mark significant patterns in nature and history.

The Hebrew calendar subsequently follows both lunar and solar cycles, with the constellations providing a framework for tracking time and marking the seasons essential to both festivals and agriculture. Celebrations like *Pesach* [Passover], *Shavuot* [Pentecost], and *Sukkot* [Tabernacles] were *moadim* ["appointed time(s)"]...*spiritual* festivals aligned with *physical* farming cycles and connected to seasons of planting, harvesting, and gratitude. Thus, God bound spiritual truths together with the practical rhythms of daily life.

Old Testament scholars like Dr. Heiser and Dr. Beale emphasize how the cosmological order showcases both God's wisdom and how natural events underscore the connections between spiritual truths and physical realities.

In essence, the twelve constellations and Hebrew months synchronize natural and spiritual rhythms, establishing the seasons as divinely ordered times for growth and community. This alignment remains significant for Messianic believers as we rediscover God's appointed times and His cycles of blessing.

However, since the Hebrew roots of the Christian faith have been forgotten for so long, we have a lot to re-learn about God's cycles of celebration. For instance...what is *Shabbat*? What is a *Rosh-Chodesh* blessing? Why do we celebrate *moadim* ["appointed time(s)"]? Remember that as followers of Yeshua, *we have been grafted into God's covenant plan with Abraham.*

Therefore, to experience the fullness of this covenant, it is essential to align with God's timing to understand when to "plant" and "harvest" in both physical and spiritual contexts. Living by these rhythms and aligning with His Word empower us to walk closely with God and enjoy His presence, further grounding our faith in the beauty of His divine order.

> **PSALM 84:5-7 CJB** | 5 How happy are those who live in your [God's] house; they never cease to praise you! 6 How happy the man whose strength is in you, in whose heart are [pilgrim] highways. 7 Passing through the [dry] Baka Valley, they make it a place of springs, and the early rain clothes it with blessings.

This journey of alignment brings the blessings of God's provision to give each of us what we truly need. By following His timing, we are brought into the rhythm of His redemptive plan and purpose...allowing us to find joy, growth, and direction in His seasons. (NOTE: Being "blessed" does not mean God gives us everything we want...it means *God always gives us what we need*).

When we yield to the gentle leading of the Holy Spirit and anchor ourselves in the truth of God's Word, we find ourselves drawn into true worship—not merely by song or ritual, but by resting in Him. In setting aside time to dwell in His presence, we align ourselves with His glory, recalibrating our hearts and minds to His purposes. In this surrender, we are positioned to advance—not by our striving, but according to His sovereign plan.

In order to experience the fullness of God's plans, our hearts and minds must be increasingly aligned with His. How do we do that? By studying, learning, and embracing the Hebrew mindset. *To that end, God designed the weeks, months, and years to bring His beloved (that's YOU!) into deeper union with Himself.*

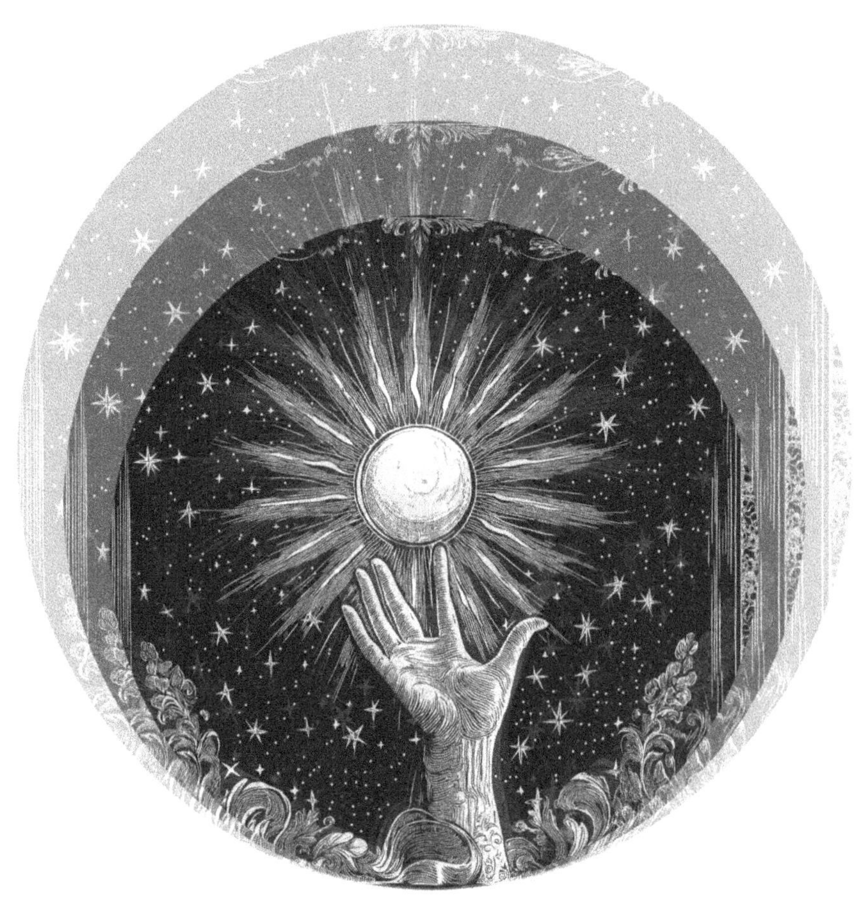

Rediscovering God's Calendar

Although the Hebrew months are identified by their numeric place on the calendar, there were occasions when they received secondary names that accompanied the number. For example, during the pre-Babylonian era, there were only four Hebrew months identified by name in Scripture:

- The first month...*Aviv* [*Nissan*]
- The second month...*Ziv* [*Iyyar*]
- The seventh month...*Eitanim* [*Tishrei*]
- The eighth month...*Bul* [*Cheshvan*]

So, why didn't the Jews retain the traditional practice of referring to months by their number?

According to the *Jerusalem Talmud* (c. 220-400 AD), modern names for the months "came up [to Israel] with [the returnees] from Babylon," at the onset of the second Jewish commonwealth in approximately 350 BC. **Nachmanides (1194-1270)**, a prominent medieval Jewish scholar, suggested that the command found in...

> **EXODUS 12:2 CJB** | [2] You are to begin your calendar with this month; it will be the first month of the year for you.

...was consistent with Jeremiah's prophecy:

> **JEREMIAH 16:14-15 CJB** | [14] "Therefore," says ADONAI, "the day will come when people will no longer swear, 'As ADONAI lives, who brought the people of Isra'el out of the land of Egypt,' [15] but, 'As ADONAI lives, who brought the people of Isra'el out of the land to the north [Babylon] and out of all the countries where he drove them'; for I will bring them back to their own land, which I gave to their ancestors."

NOTE: The month of *Nissan* was established as the "first month" because it was the month that the Hebrew people left captivity in Egypt to become the nation of Israel.

Since the original system counted the months in numeric order, starting from

Nissan, whenever someone referred to one of the months, they were, in effect, commemorating the Exodus from Egypt (e.g., "we're in the sixth month—six months since the month of the Exodus.") Thus, the numeric naming served as a constant reminder to the Jewish people that God had delivered them from slavery in Egypt (c. 1491 BC).

After God delivered Israel a second time from Babylonian captivity (c. 538 BC), the exiled Jews adopted Hebraicized forms of the Assyrian names for the months and constellations to serve as a reminder that God had redeemed them.

Rabbinical tradition explains the origin of these names:

- **Nissan** [ניסן] – The first month, referenced as *Aviv* ["spring" or "new life"] in Scripture and then renamed *Nissan*, is associated with both the spring season and the Exodus from Egypt. Its name derives from the Akkadian word *nisanu* ["start" or "beginning"].

- **Iyyar** [אייר] – The second month, referenced as *Ziv* ["radiance" or "brightness"] in Scripture (1 Kings 6:1), is linked to the blooming season since it coincides with spring and agricultural growth. Its name derives from the Akkadian word *ayaru* ["light" or "brightness"].

- **Sivan** [סיוון] – The third month is traditionally connected to the giving of the *Torah* at Mount Sinai. Its name derives from the Akkadian word *simanu* ["season" or "time"].

- **Tammuz** [תמוז] – The fourth month, named after the Babylonian deity of agriculture and fertility, is associated with tragedy (e.g., the breach of Jerusalem's walls) and is a time of mourning for the misfortunes of the Jewish people.

- **Av** [של] – The fifth month, *Av* ["father"] retains its original Hebrew meaning and is a time of national mourning, particularly for the destruction of both the First and Second Temples on the 9th of *Av* [*Tisha B'Av*]. Its name derives from the Akkadian word *abu* ["father].

- **Elul** [אלול] – The sixth month is a period of repentance and preparation for the High Holy Days of *Tishrei*. Its name derives from the Akkadian word *ululu* ["harvest"].

- **Tishrei** [תשרי] – The seventh month, referenced as *Ethanim* in Scripture and then renamed *Tishrei* after the exile, celebrates the three pilgrimage festivals (*Rosh Hashanah*, *Yom Kippur*, and *Sukkot*). Its name derives from the Akkadian word *tashritu* ["beginning"].

- **Cheshvan** [חשוון] – The eighth month, also known as *Mar-Cheshvan* due to its lack of festivals, has historical connections to the flood of Noah. Its name derives from the Akkadian word *warach-shamnu* ["eighth month"].

- **Kislev** [כסלו] – The ninth month, whose Hebrew roots form a connection to the idea of "trust" or "security", marks the season of *Hanukkah* and the onset of winter. Its name derives from the Akkadian word *kislimu* ["thickened" or "clouded"].

- **Tevet** [טבת] – The tenth month commemorates events of Jewish persecution, practices fasting, and reflects the depth of winter. Its name derives from the Akkadian word *tebitu* ["sink" or "submerge"].

- **Sh'vat** [שבט] – The eleventh month is traditionally linked to *Tu B'Sh'vat* ["New Year of Trees"] and celebrates the beginning of Israel's agricultural cycle. Its name derives from the Akkadian word *shabatu* ["strike" or "hit"] which refers to heavy rains.

- **Adar** [ענף] – The twelfth month commemorates *Purim*, a celebration of God's deliverance of the Jewish people from their enemies as recounted in the book of Esther. Its name derives from the Akkadian word *addaru* ["darkness" or "cloud"].

NOTE: Even pagan prophets, such as Balaam, used the same figures to represent the tribes (Numbers 24:7-9).

The 12 months of the Hebrew calendar correspond with both the 12 signs of the constellations and the 12 tribes of Israel. The sun, moon, and planets are like the hands of a cosmic clock and the 12 zodiac constellations represent the twelve numbers on the face of that clock. And it is this "clock" that God uses to align our lives with His purposes...*weekly, monthly, and yearly*.

> **GENESIS 1:14 CJB** | [14] God said, "Let there be lights in the dome of the sky to divide the day from the night; let them be for signs, seasons, days, and years;

When Israel abandoned God to become just like the pagan nations who worshipped false gods (i.e., the "numbers of the clock"), God sent His prophets to warn Israel that they had completely missed the point...and to *command them to stop*.

Interestingly, scholars considered the righteous Jew to be immune from the *mazzal* ["constellation" or "planet"] and offered reassurance that they need never fear any "fateful decree" of the zodiac. This view is supported by a passage in Jeremiah:

> **JEREMIAH 10:2-3 CJB** | [2] Here is what ADONAI says: "Don't learn the way of the Goyim [pagans], don't be frightened by astrological signs, even if the Goyim are afraid of them; [3] for the customs of the peoples are nothing. [...]."

This is also one of the primary reasons why the Jews were instructed NOT to consult with astrologers or rely upon their predictions:

> **DEUTERONOMY 18:11 CJB** | [11] There must not be found among you anyone who makes his son or daughter pass through fire, a diviner, a soothsayer, an enchanter, a sorcerer, a spell-caster, a consulter of ghosts or spirits, or a necromancer. For whoever does these things is detestable to ADONAI, and because of these abominations ADONAI your God is driving them out ahead of you.

In the second chapter of Numbers, the twelve tribes were divided into four camps that were assigned to four directions that corresponded to four constellations evenly spaced around a circle...just like the four points of a compass. The illustration on the following page shows the marching order of the twelve tribes of Israel...

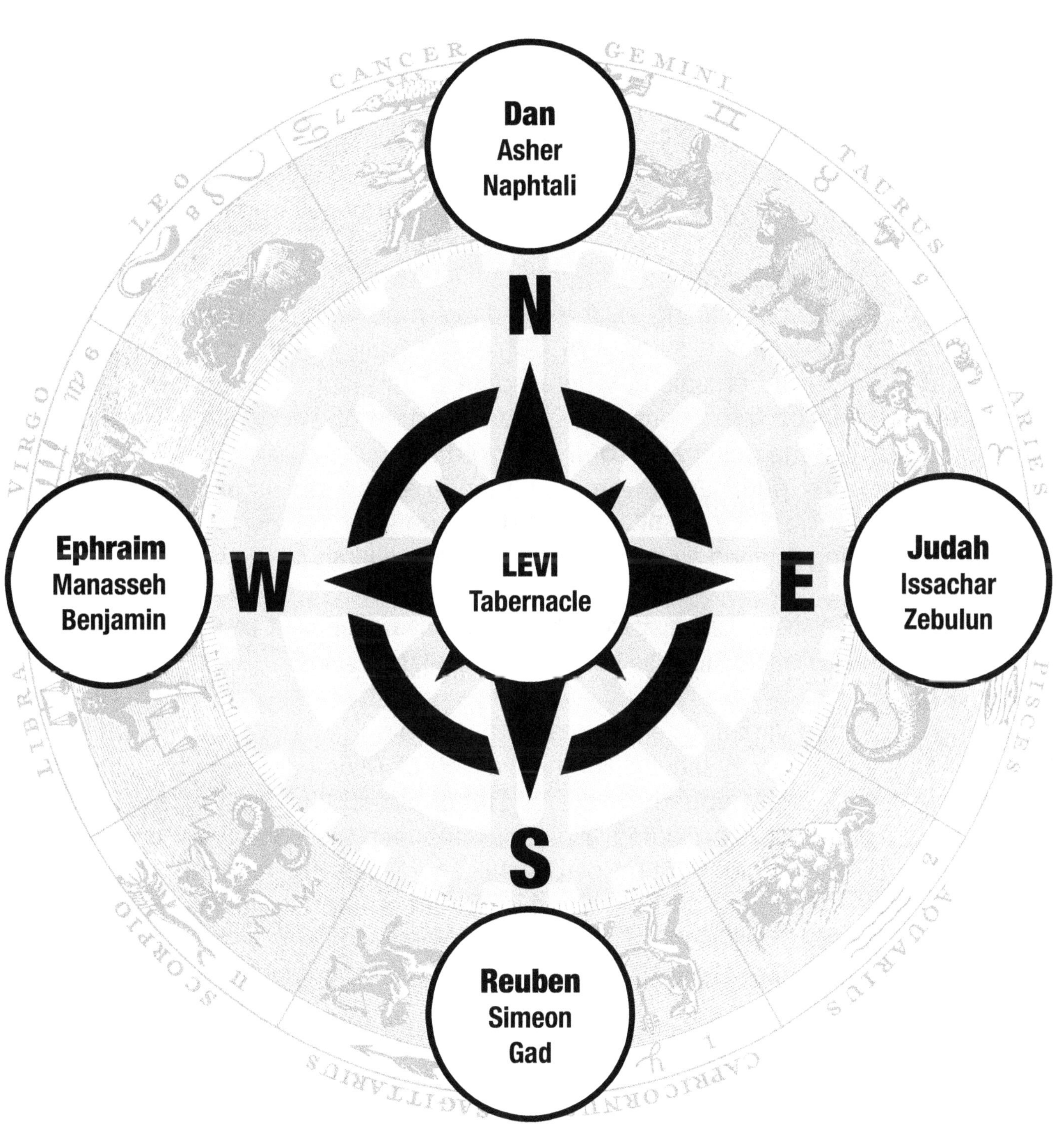
CANCER
GEMINI
TAURUS
ARIES
PISCES
AQUARIUS
CAPRICORNUS
SAGITTARIUS
SCORPIO
LIBRA
VIRGO
LEO
Dan
Asher
Naphtali
N
Ephraim
Manasseh
Benjamin
W
LEVI
Tabernacle
E
Judah
Issachar
Zebulun
S
Reuben
Simeon
Gad

The constellations also represent two important symbols/ideas: (1) *creation* and (2) the coming *Messiah*.

1. In Creation...

- **Aries** symbolized light while **Taurus** symbolized darkness.
- **Gemini** symbolized the two sexes.
- **Cancer** symbolized man, who first retreats into crevices and corners like the crab but eventually becomes as brave as a lion (**Leo**).
- **Virgo** symbolized marriage.
- **Libra** symbolized weighing all the deeds of man, who, if found guilty, was punished by **Scorpio**, a symbol of Gehinnom (Valley of the son of Hinnom, located south of Jerusalem, where some of the kings of Judah sacrificed their children by fire. Thereafter, it was deemed to be cursed. In rabbinic literature, it is the destination of the wicked).
- However, after purification in mercy, man is shot forth as an arrow from a bow, symbolized by **Sagittarius**, and becomes as innocent as a child through being purified as by water poured by **Aquarius**.

2. The Jewish Festivals demonstrated the predestined alignment of Sabbaths during which the Messiah would fulfill the following constellatory signs.

- **Virgo** [Mary the Virgin]. She was ready to give birth.
- **Libra** [The Scale or Balance]. The new moon of *Tishrei* aligned the full moon of the Lunar High Sabbath of *Sukkot* [Tabernacles] with the regular 7th day Solar Sabbath, thus providing "Balance" between the Solar and Lunar year.
- **Scorpio** [The Scorpion's Sting of Death]. The Messiah's heel rested on the head of the Scorpion and the Sting of Death would bruise the heel of the Messiah at his crucifixion.
- **Ophiuchus** [Serpent-Bearer]. The Messiah would crush the head of the Serpent at his resurrection.

Unfortunately, the zodiac constellations have been grossly perverted by occultists into astrological practices. Consequently, believers often seek to avoid the subject entirely...but the rich meaning found in these constellations behooves us to go deeper into the beauty of their biblical meaning.

For example, consider Joseph's dream of the sun, moon, and eleven stars (constellations?). In his dream, they all bowed down to him (Genesis 37:9).

When Joseph described the dream to his family, they immediately understood the eleven stars represented his eleven brothers. Was that simply because of the number eleven...or could it have been because they already understood each brother was connected to a different zodiac constellation? Historical evidence confirms that most of their names are closely connected to these constellations.

Scripture consistently portrays creation—heaven and earth alike—as ordered around the throne of God. In Psalm 19:1 CJB, the heavens *"declare the glory of God, the dome of the sky speaks the work of his hands"*, not as instruments of occultic divination, but as witnesses to His kingship.

Within this biblical worldview, several recurring patterns emerge that unite Israel's tribal structure, temple theology, prophetic vision, and even the ordered heavens themselves. Central among these is the fourfold pattern of the *man*, *lion*, *ox*, and *eagle*.

Tribal Blessings And Creation Imagery

Consider that when Jacob blessed his twelve sons (i.e., the twelve tribes), and then many years later when Moses blessed those twelve tribes...*several clear references were made to zodiac constellations*. Moreover, in Jacob's final blessing of his sons in Genesis 49:1 CJB, he was explicitly prophetic: *"Gather yourselves together, and I will tell you what will happen to you in the acharit-hayamim ["the end of the days"]."*

His words employ animal and creation imagery that signal rulership and destiny rather than mere metaphor. Reuben, as firstborn, is addressed as the embodiment of human strength and leadership (Genesis 49:3). Judah is named a *lion*, a clear emblem of kingship and authority (Genesis 49:9-10). Joseph receives a blessing framed by heaven-and-earth language—fruitfulness, strength, and abundance flowing from *"heaven above"* and the *"deep, lying below"* (Genesis 49:22-26 CJB).

Moses reinforces these themes and most notably, likens Joseph to a powerful *ox*, which symbolized strength and dominion (Deuteronomy 33:17). This blessing once again situates the twelve tribes within a cosmic framework, invoking the ordered blessing of heaven and earth (Deuteronomy 33:13). Together, these blessings present Israel as a people formed to reflect God's creational order.

The Connection To The Four Living Creatures In Ezekiel And Revelation

This same fourfold pattern appears in the throne visions of Ezekiel and John. Ezekiel sees four living beings, each bearing the faces of a *man*, *lion*, *ox*, and *eagle* (Ezekiel 1:10). These beings function as throne guardians, later identified as *cherubim*, and are closely associated with God's glory (Ezekiel 10:1-22).

John's vision in Revelation intentionally echoes Ezekiel: *"The first living being was like a lion, the second living being was like an ox, the third living being had a face that looked human, and the fourth living being was like a flying eagle"* (Revelation 4:7 CJB).

Positioned at the center of heavenly worship, these creatures proclaim God's holiness (Revelation 4:8). As Dr. G. K. Beale notes, Revelation repeatedly draws on Old Testament temple imagery to present heaven as the true sanctuary with God as King ruling the universe.

Together, the four faces represent the fullness of animate creation under His authority:

- **Man.** Humanity as God's image-bearer and steward (Genesis 1:26-28)
- **Lion.** Wild animals and royal authority, later fulfilled in Judah and Yeshua (Genesis 49:9; Revelation 5:5)
- **Ox.** Domesticated animals, strength, service, and sacrificial labor (Deuteronomy 33:17)
- **Eagle.** The birds of the heavens, swiftness, and transcendence (Exodus 19:4; Isaiah 40:31)

The vision proclaims all of creation gathers around God's throne in worship.

The Heavens As Ordered Testimony

Scripture affirms that the stars and constellations are part of God's created order, appointed *"for signs, seasons, days, and years"* (Genesis 1:14 CJB). Or, when God challenged Job regarding the constellations to emphasize His divine sovereignty (Job 38:32). This is astronomy, *not* astrology.

In the Ancient Near East (ANE), four constellations marked the cardinal structure of the sky: *Aquarius* ["man"], *Leo* ["lion"], *Taurus* ["ox"], and *Aquila* ["eagle"]. Their correspondence with Ezekiel's and John's four living creatures reflects a shared creational order, not an occultic interpretation. The heavens, like the Temple, testify to God's divine rule.

Among Jacob's sons, four emerge as structural leaders of Israel: Reuben (man), Judah (lion), Joseph (ox), and Dan (eagle).

Reuben. As Jacob's firstborn, he is the embodiment of man's strength and dignity: *"you are my firstborn, my strength, the first fruits of my manhood"* (Genesis 49:3 CJB). Though he forfeits his status through sin (Genesis 49:4), his role reflects the human face among the four living creatures—the image-bearing representative of humanity entrusted with stewardship over creation (Genesis 1:26-28).

Judah. He is explicitly identified with the lion, symbolizing royal authority and kingship: *"Y'hudah [Judah] is a lion's cub [...] The scepter will not pass from Y'hudah" [Judah]* (Genesis 49:9-10 CJB). This imagery carries forward to its ultimate fulfillment in Yeshua, *"the Lion of the tribe of Y'hudah [Judah]"* (Revelation 5:5 CJB).

Joseph. He is most clearly associated with the ox, a symbol of strength, service, and fruitfulness. Moses explicitly uses this imagery when blessing Joseph: *"His firstborn bull — glory is his; his horns are those of a wild ox"* (Deuteronomy 33:17 CJB). Joseph's life and blessing emphasize provision and sustaining power, as he preserves Israel during famine (Genesis 50:20). His sons, Ephraim and Manasseh, later anchor the western side of Israel's camp (Numbers 2:18-24).

Dan. His connection to the eagle is more functional than explicit. Jacob describes Dan as both judge and watchful presence (Genesis 49:16-17). In the camp arrangement, Dan occupies the northern position and serves as the rear guard for Israel's movements (Numbers 2:25-31).

Biblically, the eagle represents height, vigilance, and swift oversight—imagery describing God's protection and exalted power (Exodus 19:4; Isaiah 40:31). This aligns with Dan's role as guardian and overseer within Israel's structure.

These four tribes—Reuben, Judah, Joseph, and Dan—anchor the four sides of Israel's encampment around the Tabernacle (Numbers 2). This earthly arrangement mirrors the heavenly reality revealed to Ezekiel and John as a microcosm of creation.

The meaning is neither astrological nor speculative, but a form of worship that honors God and His ordering of heaven and earth around His throne. This is why Israel was called to represent that order as *"a kingdom of cohanim [priests] for me, a nation set apart"* (Exodus 19:5-6 CJB).

This vision culminates in Yeshua, *"the Lion of the tribe of Judah"* (Revelation 5:5 CJB), in whom heaven and earth, throne and temple, creation and redemption are brought together.

> "The Bible teaches that the sun, moon and stars are positioned by God for a purpose, and He arranged them in the Heavens to establish His time in our lives.
>
> CHUCK D. PIERCE

As you begin to discover God's purpose for each month, pray that...

- He will help you develop a "Hebrew mindset."
- He will help you establish new patterns of weekly, monthly, and yearly cycles of alignment.
- He will strengthen your trust in His power, love, and mercy.
- He will demolish any false agreements that you have made and restore you into His Truth.

ALIGNING WITH THE HEBREW CALENDAR

The Hebrew calendar is based on both the moon (lunar) and the sun (solar). Each month begins with the new moon, but because a lunar cycle lasts about 29½ days, Hebrew months cannot all be the same length. As a result, months alternate between 29 and 30 days.

In biblical times, the start of a new month—called *Rosh Chodesh* ["Head of the Month"]—was declared by the *Sanhedrin* (Israel's highest rabbinical court) based on testimony from witnesses who had seen the first crescent of the new moon. For this reason, the *Sanhedrin* gathered on the 30th day of each month in expectation of the new month beginning.

If witnesses confirmed the new moon on that day, the previous month ended with 29 days, and the 30th day became the first day of the new month. If no confirmation was given, the previous month was counted 30 days, and the new month began the following day. This is why *Rosh Chodesh* lasts either one or two days. In other words:

- If the previous month has 30 days, *Rosh Chodesh* is observed for two days: the 30th day of the old month and the 1st day of the new month.
- If the previous month has 29 days, *Rosh Chodesh* is observed for one day only: the 1st day of the new month.

Due to this pattern: *Cheshvan*, *Iyyar*, *Tammuz*, *Elul*, and *Adar* (including *Adar II* in leap years) always have two days of *Rosh Chodesh*.

Tishrei, *Sh'vat*, *Nissan*, *Sivan*, and *Av* always have one day of *Rosh Chodesh*.

However, *Kislev* and *Tevet* vary from year to year. In some years, both have one day of *Rosh Chodesh*; in others, both have two days; and in some years, *Kislev* has one day while *Tevet* has two.

This flexibility allows the Hebrew calendar to remain aligned with both the lunar cycle and the solar year, preserving the rhythm of the biblical festivals within their appointed seasons.

Sabbath: God's Design For The Week

God's life cycles are designed to elevate our spiritual walk into a deeper level of connection with Him. We are meant to experience God's presence and to live a meaningful life. But this does not happen by creating and following meaningless rituals. Instead, following God's cycles of life authentically and consistently produces blessing. Thus, the practice of a weekly rhythm of *Shabbat* ["Sabbath"] trains us in wisdom and discernment...as we develop spiritually healthy boundaries for ourselves and for our families.

Maturing in our faith requires us to set a Spirit-led perimeter around our hearts, our families, our time…and then standing firm.

God Himself modeled this weekly cycle of rest at the creation of the world. Although He promised great blessings to those who kept His Sabbath holy…it can seem so difficult to set aside even one day to simply rest and enjoy His goodness.

So, what can we do on the Sabbath? Anything and nothing. When Yeshua saw how the Pharisees were burdening the people with religious protocols concerning the Sabbath...he was devastated. Because the true purpose of the Sabbath is to *enjoy the ultimate blessing…God's presence*.

To do this, we set aside time, from sundown to sundown, to release the burdens of our life to God and rest in Him. It is an act of worship meant to help us regularly experience physical and spiritual renewal in union with Him.

> "Sabbath is a time consecrated to enjoy what is beautiful and good...a time to light candles, sing songs, worship, tell stories, bless our children, give thanks, share meals, nap, and even make love. It is a time to be nourished and refreshed as we let our work, our chores and our important projects lie fallow, trusting that there are larger forces at work taking care of the world while we are at rest.
>
> WAYNE MULLER

COLOSSIANS 2:16-17 CJB | [16] So don't let anyone pass judgment on you in connection with eating and drinking, or in regard to a Jewish festival or Rosh-Hodesh [head of the month] or Shabbat [Sabbath]. [17] These are a shadow of things that are coming, but the body is of the Messiah.

There are many Christians who offer this passage as theological proof that the New Testament Church eliminated the Sabbath. The word "judge" means "to pronounce an opinion concerning right and wrong" (*Thayer's Lexicon*). In several translations the word "is" in verse 17 is italicized which indicates that it was absent from the original Greek text and later added by translators.

In verse 16, Paul warns believers against allowing others to determine the "right or wrong" way to observe these sacred festivals. Instead, these matters should be determined by the Messianic community in accordance with the Scriptures (that plainly teach the Sabbath should be observed).

Moreover, consider the implications of verse 17, *"These are a shadow of things that are coming, but the body is of the Messiah."* A shadow cannot be separated from its object. For example, the shadow of a tree leads directly back to the tree. If you remove the tree, *there is no shadow*. Therefore, if the Sabbath is a shadow of things to come—God's eternal rest—then why would it be taken away? Yet, that is exactly what many Christians suggest should be done.

Perhaps this erroneous reasoning stems from newer Bible translations that often attach negative connotations to the word "shadow" in order to highlight the supremacy of Jesus. All that matters is Jesus, they say. Ignore his example—just believe in him. But both aspects are important and neither diminish even one iota of Jesus' supremacy.

One final point of interest is that Paul wrote this letter to the *Gentiles* at Colossi. Before joining the Messianic community, these *Gentiles* had never observed God's Sabbath command or celebrated His festivals. Yet, Paul instructs them not to *"let anyone pass judgment on you in connection with eating and drinking, or in regard to a Jewish festival or Rosh-Hodesh or Shabbat."*

Why would he say this to *Gentiles*, since they had never followed the *Torah* nor observed its laws or practices in the first place? *Because God still wants His family of believers, Jew and Gentile alike, to remain connected to the heart behind these observances and celebrations.*

> **1 CORINTHIANS 12:27 CJB** | [27] Now you together [Jew and Gentile] constitute the body of the Messiah, and individually you are parts of it.

> **COLOSSIANS 2:13 CJB** | [13] And you, who were dead in your trespasses and the uncircumcision of your flesh, God made alive together with him, having forgiven us all our trespasses [...]

Additionally, it is an almost certainty that those "passing judgement" were *Jews* whose cultural and spiritual heritage was based on *Torah* directives concerning eating, drinking, Jewish festivals, *Rosh-Hodesh* celebrations, and *Shabbat*.

ALIGNING WITH THE SABBATH

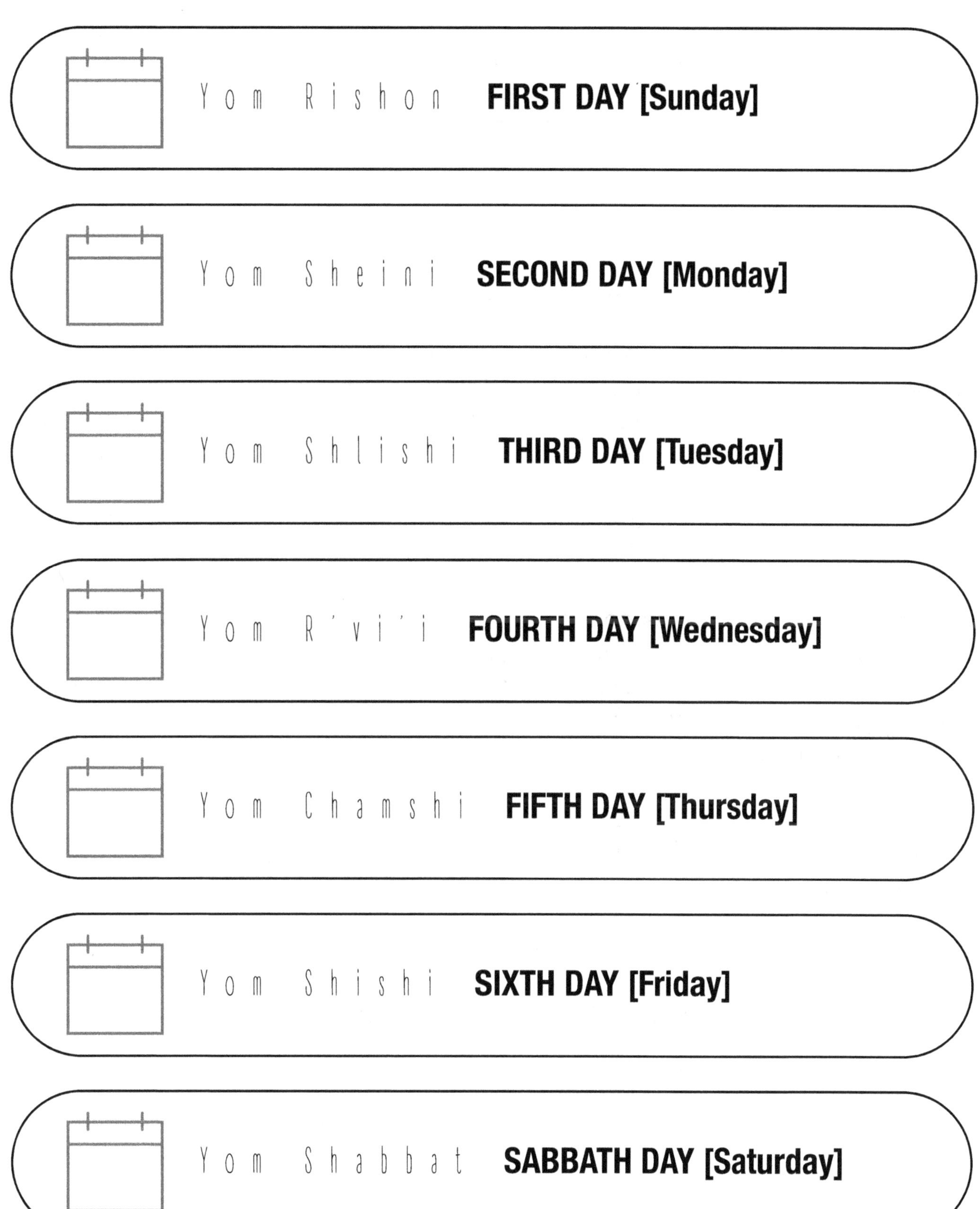

Rosh Chodesh: God's Design For The Month

> **NUMBERS 28:11-13 CJB** | 11 "'At each Rosh-Hodesh of yours, you are to present a burnt offering to ADONAI consisting of two young bulls, one ram and seven male lambs in their first year and without defect; 12 with six quarts of fine flour mixed with olive oil as a grain offering for the one ram; 13 and two quarts of fine flour mixed with olive oil as a grain offering for each lamb. This will be the burnt offering giving a fragrant aroma, an offering made by fire for ADONAI.

Traditionally, the new moon (*Rosh-Chodesh*) was a monthly reminder to set apart time to honor God with the "first-fruits" (Leviticus 23:10) of your life and to offer gratitude for His blessings. God established these regular cycles of "sabbathing" to help us develop a first-fruits mindset in every area of our lives.

This means offering God the first-fruits of our attention…our time…and our money…all of which honors Him and releases His blessing.

In fact, our Creator desires connection with us so much, that He declared one day a week (*Shabbat*) and the first day of each month (*Rosh-Chodesh*) be spent in communion with Him. When we honor these *moadim* ["appointed time(s)"], we are declaring (with our actions) that we joyfully celebrate Him before anything else.

This principle still applies today. As we honor God with the *first* of our time…*all* of our time is set-apart (made special or holy) and we are positioned to walk in His presence all month!

In Yeshua's day, *Rosh-Chodesh* was an important celebration for God's people. When the first sliver of a new moon appeared in the sky, it marked the beginning of a new month which meant that a jubilant celebration was about to take place!

Thus, the first day of the Hebrew month is set apart…*just like a Sabbath*. So, what can we do on *Rosh-Chodesh*? Again, anything and nothing. Talk with your family (or just yourself) about how to celebrate the Sabbath of the new month.

Remember, this is *not* about following empty religious rituals or box-checking "spiritual" activities, it's about *intentionally setting aside the first-fruits of your time to connect with God and rest in His presence*.

I like to think of it as a date with God, a time to connect with my family, to enjoy each others company, and to remember the blessings we have been given. We make *challah* bread, eat a communion meal together, and generally have fun.

Find things you enjoy doing as a family and CELEBRATE!!!

And someday we will all celebrate *Rosh-Chodesh* together...

> **ISAIAH 66:23 CJB** | 23 "Every month on Rosh-Chodesh and every week on Shabbat [Sabbath], everyone living will come to worship in my presence," says ADONAI.

What an amazing picture! In the new heaven and earth, all those who love God, both Jew and Gentile, will come together to worship in His presence.

[NOTE: Traditionally, *Rosh-Chodesh* also honors women, as noted in the Talmudic commentary, *Ba'alei Tosafot* by Rashi (1040-1105), an influential French rabbi. The women of Israel earned this distinction because they refused to contribute their jewelry for the construction of the golden calf.

A traditional prayer for *Rosh-Chodesh*…

ברוך אתה ה' אלוהינו מלך העולם אשר נתן את ימי ראש חודש לעמו ישראל לזכור.

TRANSLITERATION: Baruch a-toh A-do-noi Elo-hei-nu me-lech ha-o-lam she-na-san ro-shei cho-da-shim le-a-mo yis-ra-el le-zi-ka-ron.

TRANSLATION: Blessed are You, LORD our God, King of the universe, who has given the days of Rosh-Chodesh to His people Israel for remembrance.

ALIGNING WITH THE ROSH-CHODESH

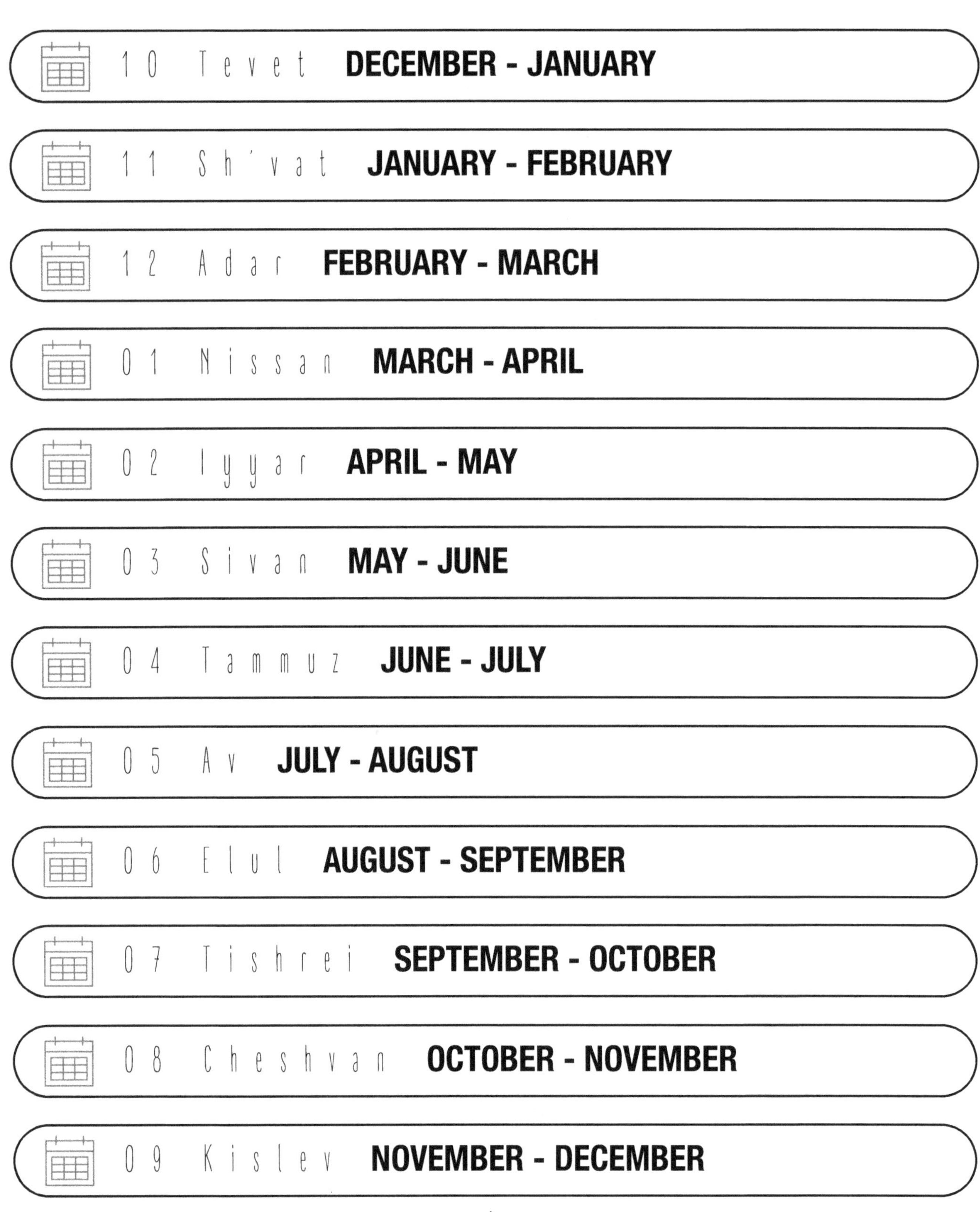

שלום

ALIGNING WITH THE ROSH-CHODESH

Quick reminder: *Rosh-Chodesh* ["first-fruits"] is the first day of every month and is celebrated as a Sabbath day...EXCEPT for the months that contain 30 days. Those months (*Adar*, *Iyyar*, *Tammuz*, *Elul*, and *Cheshvan*) celebrate a "double Sabbath."

God established these monthly/yearly cycles because He knows we need to "E.A.T." (Effort.Alignment.Timing) in order to thrive in His design.

לחגוג

DAYS OF ROSH-CHODESH FOR 2026 (5786)

11 Sh'vat | Jan 18-19

12 Adar | Feb 16-18

01 Nissan | Mar 18-19

02 Iyyar | Apr 16-18

03 Sivan | May 16-17

04 Tammuz | Jun 14-16

05 Av | Jul 14-15

06 Elul | Aug 12-14

07 Tishrei | Sep 11-13*

08 Cheshvan | Oct 10-12

09 Kislev | Nov 9-11

10 Tevet | Dec 9-11

HIGH HOLY DAYS FOR 2026 (5786)

Purim	Mar 2-3 | Adar 14
Pesach [Passover]	Apr 1-9 | Nissan 15-22
Counting the Omer	Apr 2-May 20 | Nissan 16-Sivan 5
Shav'uot [Pentecost]	May 21-23 | Sivan 6-7
***Rosh Hashanah [Head of the Year]**	Sep 11-13 | Tishrei 1-2
Yom Kippur [Day of Atonement]	Sep 20-21 | Tishrei 10
Sukkot [Feast of Tabernacles]	Sep 25-Oct 2 | Tishrei 15-21
Hanukkah [Festival of Lights]	Dec 4-12 | Kislev 25-Tevet 2

*Since it coincides with Rosh Hashanah, it is "combined" with the holiday instead.

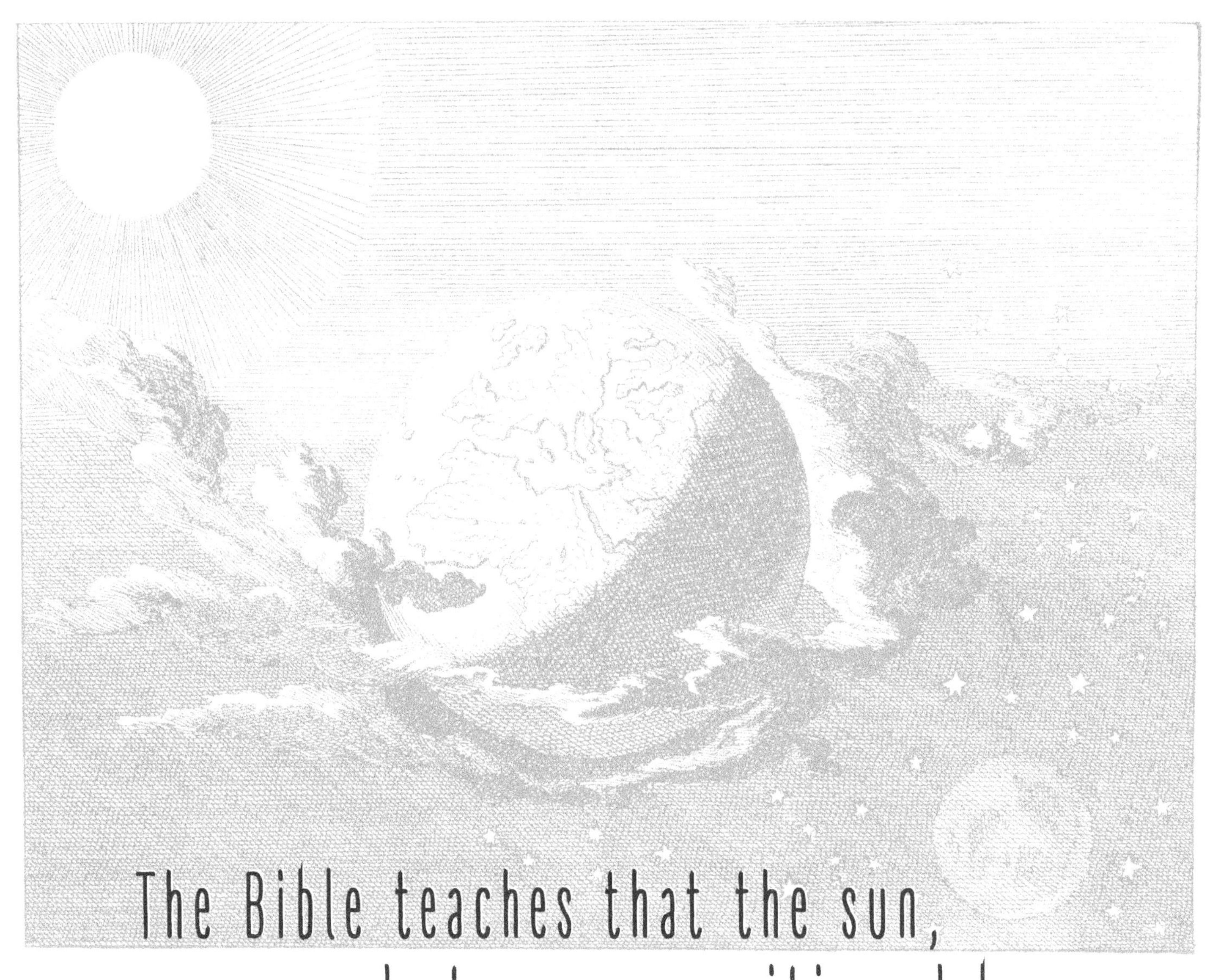

The Bible teaches that the sun, moon, and stars are positioned by God for a purpose, and He arranged them in the Heavens to establish His time in our lives.

CHUCK D. PIERCE

THRIVING IN THE SEASONS

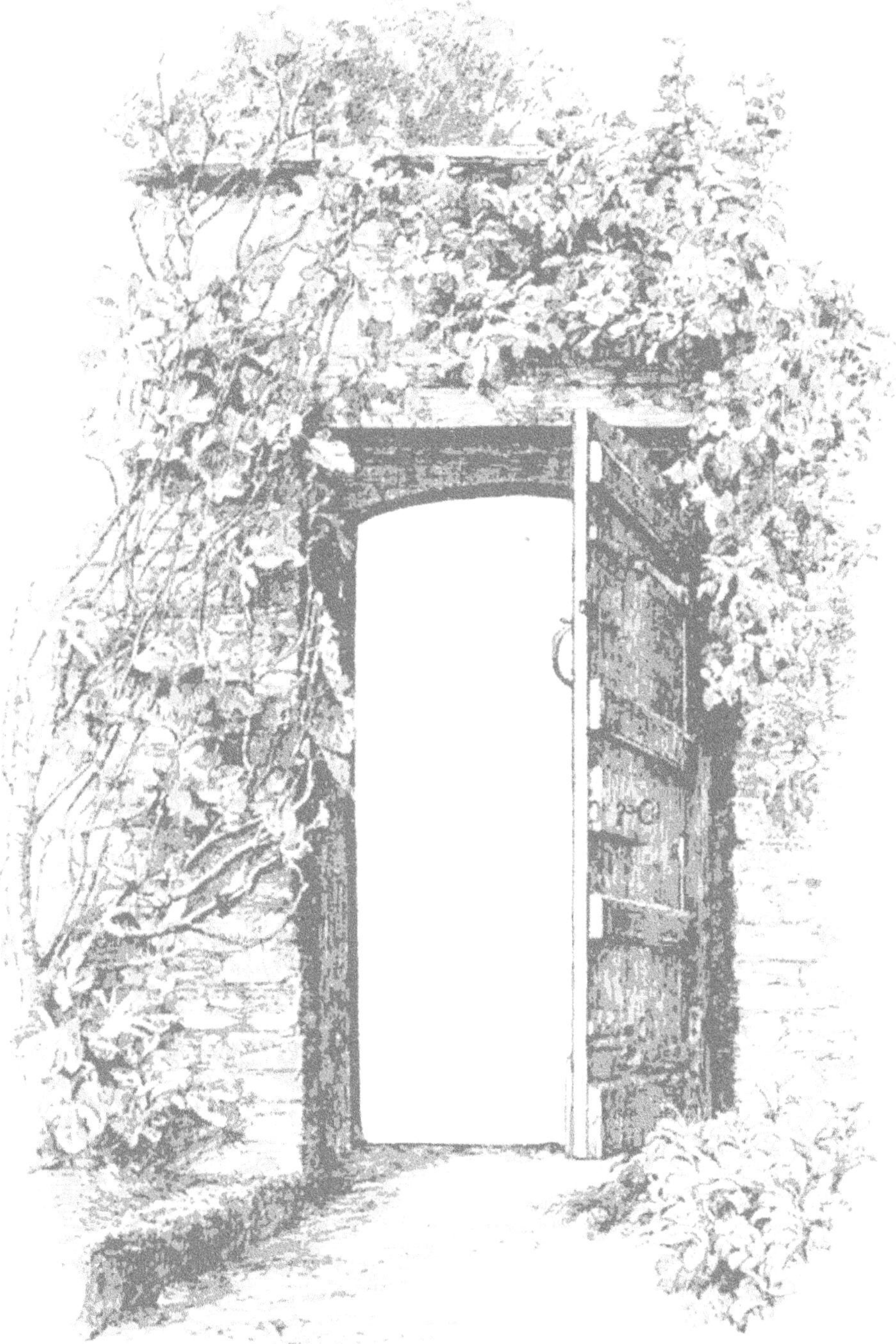

Part 4

THRIVING IN THE SEASONS

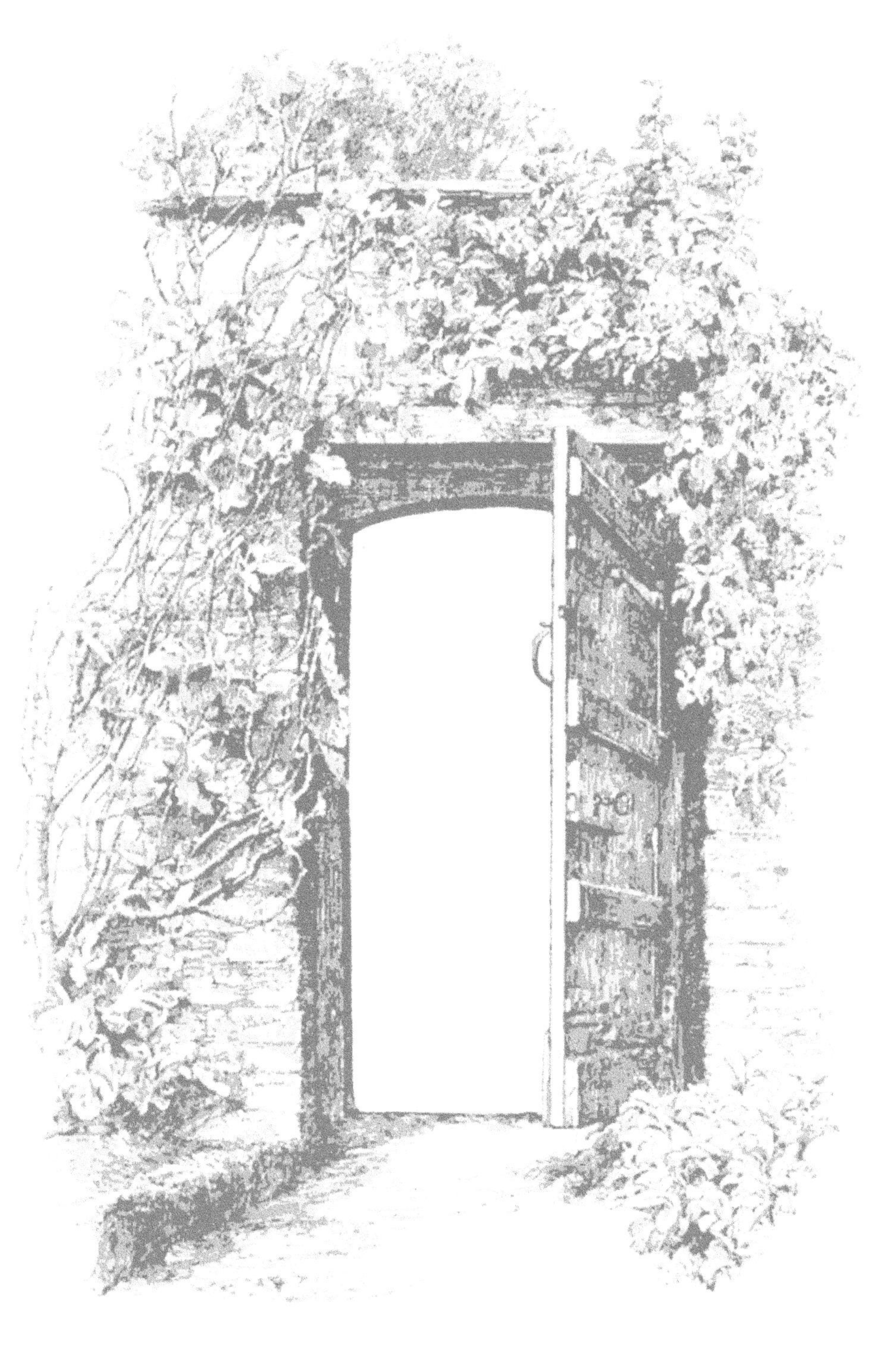

Part 4

THE HEBREW MONTHS

Daily life in ancient Israel (and everywhere else for that matter) was largely influenced by things beyond human control...namely the seasons and the weather. Thus, God created the seasons to teach us that (1) He controls the timing of events, and (2) His promises are always true.

God divided a year into four seasons: Winter, Spring, Summer, and Autumn. The function of these natural weather cycles physically illustrate the spiritual process of aligning our minds, hearts, and actions with His design in order to experience the reward of His intimate presence.

> **GENESIS 8:22 CJB** | 22 So long as the earth exists, sowing time and harvest, cold and heat, summer and winter, and day and night will not cease.

A *natural* season represents one of the four major divisions of the calendar year and is determined by the earth's yearly revolution around the SUN...but a *spiritual* season depends on the extent to which our lives revolve around the SON.

> **ECCLESIASTES 3:1 CJB** | 1 For everything there is a season, a right time for every intention under heaven –

> **PSALM 104:19 CJB** | 19 You [ADONAI] made the moon to mark the seasons, and the sun knows when to set.

> **DANIEL 2:21 CJB** | 21 he [ADONAI] brings the changes of seasons and times; he installs and deposes kings; he gives wisdom to the wise and knowledge to those with discernment.

The Scriptures only recognize Summer and Winter by name, or as the writers of the Talmud put it, "the days of sun" and "the days of rain."

- Autumn [Heb. *stav*] is only mentioned once (Song of Solomon 2:11)...as a reference to the time of winter rains.
- Spring [Heb. *aviv*] is mentioned twice, and both instances denote a stage in the ripening of barley rather than a particular season. Barley ripens during the "season" of *Aviv* [*hodesh ha'aviv*] and this occurs during the Hebrew month of *Nissan*.

But the four seasons also serve a spiritual purpose. In *The Screwtape Letters*, C. S. Lewis imagines a correspondence between a chief demonic tempter named Screwtape and his apprentice, Wormwood. At one point, Screwtape comments on "*the horror of the Same Old Thing.*"

According to the demon, the familiarity bred of contempt is, "*one of the most valuable passions we have produced in the human heart—an endless source of heresies in religion, folly in counsel, infidelity in marriage, and inconstancy in friendship.*"

Screwtape further explains: "*The humans live in time, and experience reality successively. To experience much of it, therefore, they must experience many different things; in other words, they must experience change. And since they need change, the Enemy [Screwtape's name for God]...has made change pleasurable to them, just as He has made eating pleasurable. But since He does not wish them to make change, any more than eating, an end in itself, He has balanced the love of change in them by a love of permanence. He has contrived to gratify both tastes together in the very world He has made, by that union of change and permanence which we call Rhythm.*"

Consequently, "*He [God] gives them the seasons, each season different yet every year the same, so that spring is always felt as a novelty yet always as the recurrence of an immemorial theme.*"

Lewis has got it exactly right: we're glad its spring...but we're also glad that it's *not always* spring. In this way, each season illustrates the beauty of the Great Designer who created the seasons.

The Jews, influenced by Greco-Roman civilization, later divided the year into four seasons, naming each according to the original Hebrew name of the month in which the season began:

- WINTER | *Tevet*
- SPRING | *Nissan*
- SUMMER | *Tammuz*
- AUTUMN | *Tishrei*

WINTER ➪ SPRING ➪ SUMMER ➪ AUTUMN

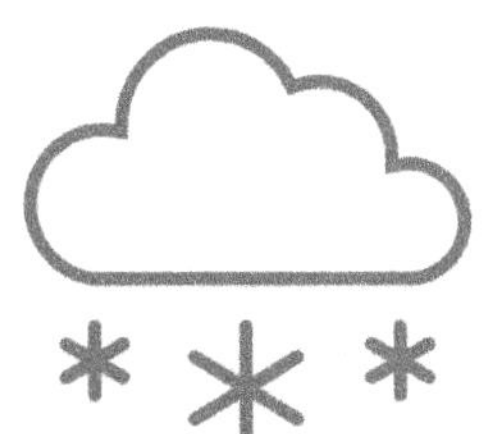

WINTER | **Tevet**

10 Tevet | December – January
11 Sh'vat | January – February
12 Adar | February – March

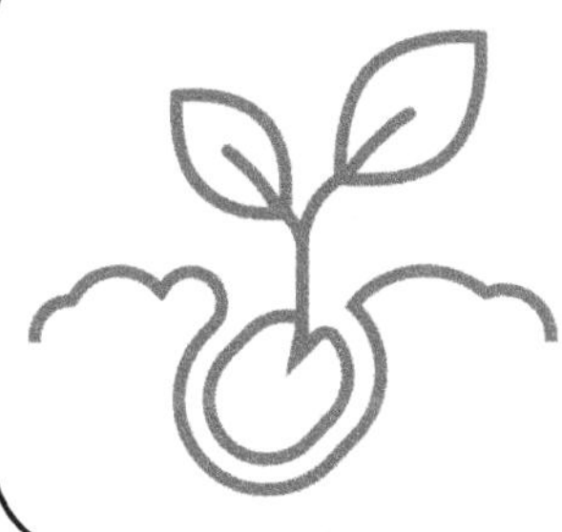

SPRING | **Nissan**

1 Nissan | March – April
2 Iyyar | April – May
3 Sivan | May – June

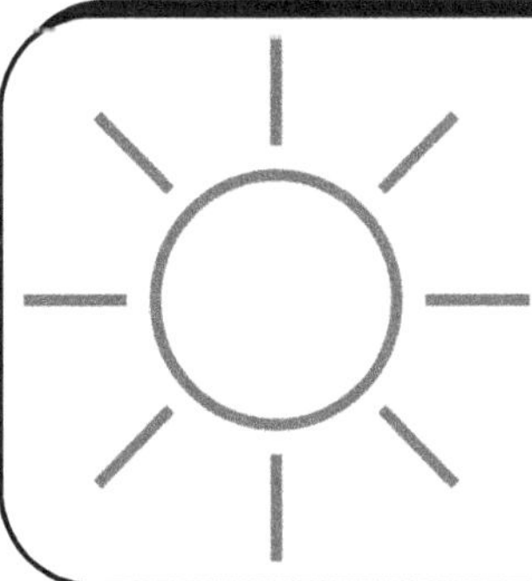

SUMMER | **Tammuz**

4 Tammuz | June – July
5 Av | July – August
6 Elul | August – September

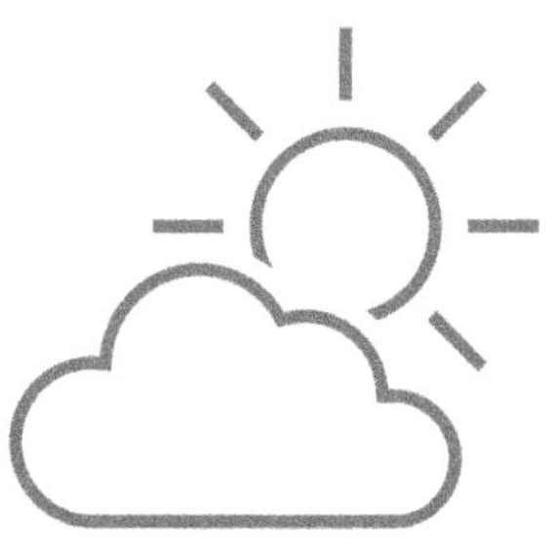

AUTUMN | **Tishrei**

7 Tishrei | September – October
8 Cheshvan | October – November
9 Kislev | November – December

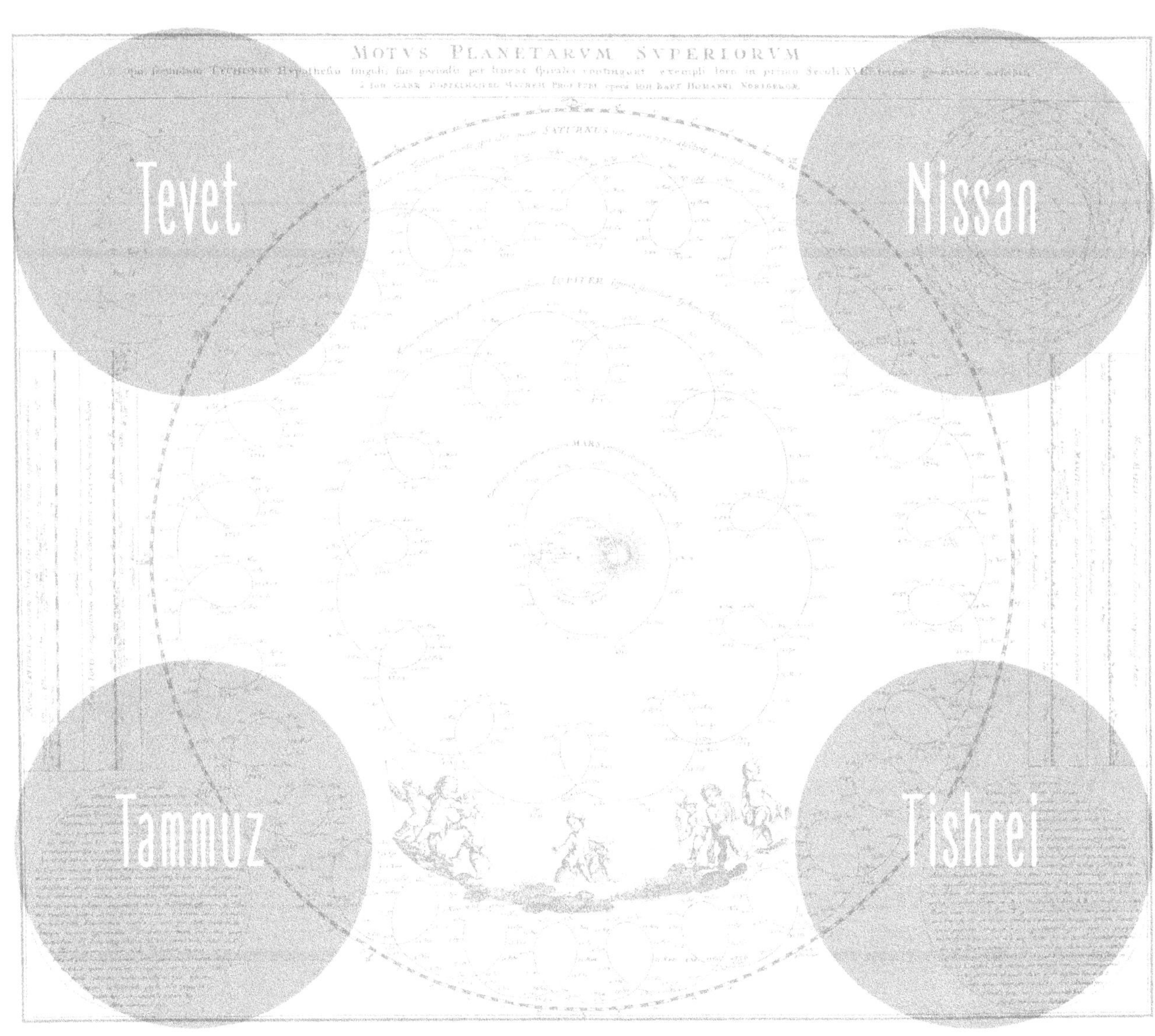
MOTVS PLANETARVM SVPERIORVM
Tevet
Nissan
SATURNUS
IUPITER
MARS
Tammuz
Tishrei

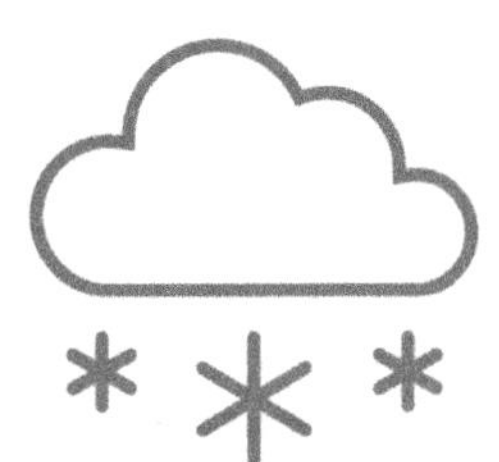

WINTER | **Tevet**

10 Tevet | December – January
11 Sh'vat | January – February
12 Adar | February – March

Winter [Heb. Choref]. This is a season of dormancy and preparation. Agriculturally, winter in Israel is the season of "early rains" which are essential for softening the ground in preparation for planting. The rains symbolize God's provision (Deuteronomy 11:14) when the early and late rains were promised as part of His blessing for obedience.

Spiritually, winter is a time of waiting and dependence on God. It is a season of reflection, allowing for spiritual restoration as the land lies dormant. Marty Solomon of the BEMA Podcast describes how times of apparent stillness are (1) essential for growth and (2) preparation for future fruitfulness, all of which is powerfully illustrated in the agricultural rhythm of the winter season.

Historically, the Jewish festival of Hanukkah, which celebrates the rededication of the Temple, takes place in winter, representing hope and light in the midst of darkness. According to Dr. Michael S. Heiser, the symbolic significance of light in biblical theology demonstrates God's presence and guidance during challenging times. Thus, winter is a period to reflect on God's faithfulness and prepare for future growth.

10 Tevet ["sinking" or "immersing"] • **11 Sh'vat** ["new year for trees"] • **12 Adar** ["almonds blooming"]

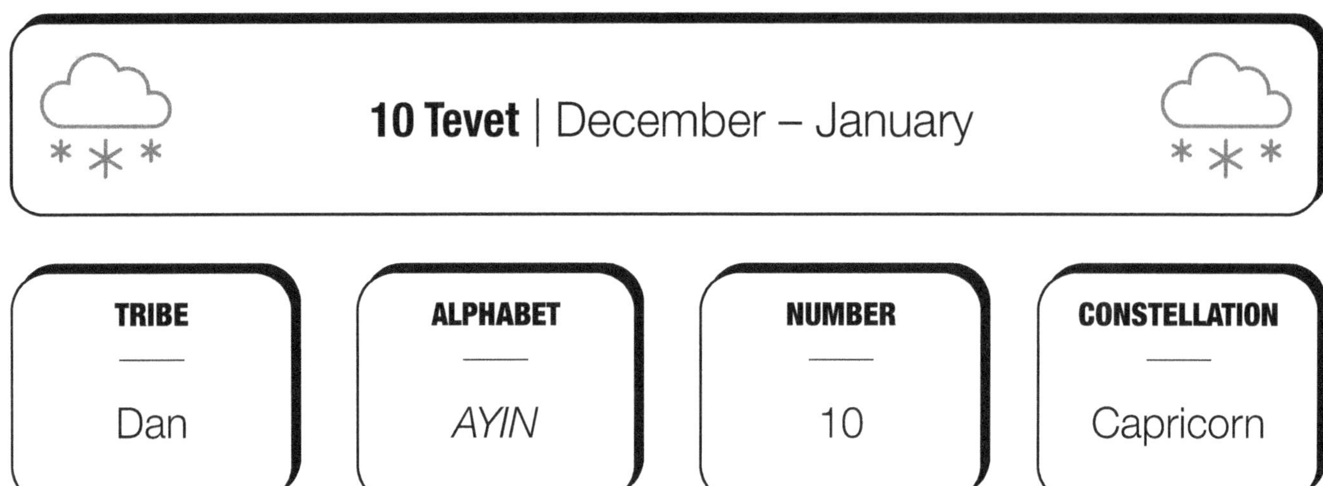

Jacob + Bilhah = Dan

GENESIS 30:4-6 CJB | 4 So she [Rachel] gave him Bilhah her slave-girl as his wife, and Ya'akov [Jacob] went in and slept with her. 5 Bilhah conceived and bore Ya'akov a son. 6 Rachel said, "God has judged in my favor; indeed, he has heard me and given me a son." Therefore, she called him Dan [he judged].

The Blessing Of Jacob…

GENESIS 49:16-18 CJB | 16 "Dan will judge his people as one of the tribes of Isra'el. 17 Dan will be a viper on the road, a horned snake in the path that bites the horse's heels, so its rider falls off backward. 18 I wait for your deliverance, ADONAI.

The Blessing Of Moses…

DEUTERONOMY 33:22 CJB | 22 Of Dan he said: "Dan is a lion cub leaping forth from Bashan."

Historical and biblical context. The month of *Tevet* holds a number of sorrowful historical associations for the Jewish people. The 10th of *Tevet* marks a fast day, *Asarah B'Tevet,* which commemorates the siege of Jerusalem by Nebuchadnezzar, and ultimately led to the destruction of the First Temple in 586 BC (2 Kings 25:1-2; Jeremiah 52:4-5).

[NOTE: This event marks the beginning of the Hebrew exile to Babylon].

Tevet is also connected to the book of Esther. It was during the month of *Tevet* when Esther was presented to King Ahasuerus and ultimately became queen (Esther 2:16-17). This association links the month to themes of divine providence and hidden deliverance.

The tribe of Dan. *Tevet* is traditionally connected to the tribe of Dan, one of the twelve sons of Jacob, and had a mixed reputation in Scripture, being both praised for its strength and condemned for its idolatry (Judges 18:30-31).

Dan is often associated with judgment and discernment, which can be reflected in the introspective nature of the fasts that occur during the month. The tribe's emblem is the serpent, a symbol of cunning, shrewdness, and protection, which also highlights the need for vigilance during times of spiritual trial.

The letter Ayin. *Tevet* is associated with the Hebrew letter *Ayin* ["eye"] and can symbolize insight, perception, and judgment. The letter also represents seeing beyond the surface to understand deeper truths and perceive what might not be readily apparent.

This interpretation aligns with the larger biblical themes of *Tevet*, particularly the hiddenness of God's work in the story of Esther, where providence was at work behind the scenes.

The number ten. *Tevet*, as the tenth month of the Hebrew calendar, is associated number ten (10) which represents completeness or divine order. Both the Ten Commandments and the ten plagues loosed upon Egypt are examples of this completeness. As the tenth month, *Tevet* serves as a time of completing the spiritual work of judgment and refinement initiated earlier in the Hebrew year, such as during *Yom Kippur* ["Day of Atonement"] and *Sukkot* ["Feast of Tabernacles"].

The constellation Capricorn. *Tevet* is associated with the constellation of Capricorn [Heb. *Gedi*] and is represented by a goat or young lamb. In Hebrew tradition, goats were used for offerings and sacrifices (Leviticus 16:10) which symbolized the bearing of sin and atonement.

The constellation reflects themes of judgment, atonement, and the ongoing need for spiritual purification and reflection. While the stars are not heavily emphasized in traditional Jewish scholarship, the zodiacal symbolism often parallels the introspective and penitential mood of the month.

Spiritual focus of Tevet. For followers of Yeshua, the Hebrew month of *Tevet* offers us a priceless opportunity for spiritual reflection, judgment, and hope. It is a time to remember the reality of exile, both physical and spiritual, and to rejoice in the restoration that Yeshua brings.

The themes of discernment, hiddenness, and divine providence remind us that God is always at work...even when His hand is not immediately visible. *Tevet* encourages a deepened reliance on Yeshua's atonement for our sins and the completeness of His redemptive work which offers us both spiritual cleansing and the hope of full restoration in the age to come.

The month serves to remind us of our need for vigilance, discernment, and hope in the face of adversity, and it invites us to trust in God's providence, even when hidden from view.

Alignment in Tevet. The reason we process each month is to remain in alignment with God's rhythm of life. This means that we fearlessly examine both the good and the bad that happened each month to know where to invite God for healing, encouragement, direction, blessing, or repentance.

We believe that *unresolved grief is undelivered communication of an emotional nature.* When these communications (either positive or negative) are identified and expressed...*we experience emotional completion*. This enables us to keep our our hearts *clear* and *connected* as we practice alignment with God...instead of carrying our wounds and burdens into the next month.

Here's how we're going to use the Graphing Tool on the following pages:

STEP NO. 1: On the graph, start at the **BEGINNING OF MONTH** and continue to the **END OF MONTH**...

- Write down any events that happened, with positive events above the line and negative events below the line.
- Draw a line to represent the intensity of the event (the longer the line, the greater the intensity).
- Label each event with one of these emotional components:
  A = Apology • F = Forgive • S = Significant Emotional Statement

STEP NO. 2: Write out a **Significant Emotional Statement** for each event. This represents your emotional truth about how this event affected you. Some events can also have an **Apology** or a **Forgive** included in the statement and might be addressed to God, to another person, or even to yourself.

Reflect on the past month and write out (1) anything you need to apologize for, (2) anything you need to forgive, and (3) anything that describes your emotional truth. (Remember there is no judgment here...this is just for your heart to be clear, so be honest!)

STEP NO. 3: Write down anything that comes to your mind when you reflect on how God has shown up in these events.

In our monthly *Zoom Coaching* call, Inspired Life members will read their sentences and connections to their partner.

THE HEBREW MONTHS

END OF MONTH

STEP NO. 1

A = Apologies • F = Forgives • SES = Positive Significant Emotional Statements

Positive is above the line | **Negative** is below the line

BEGINNING OF MONTH

STEP NO. 2

A = Apologies

F = Forgives

SES = Positive Significant Emotional Statements

STEP NO. 3

REFLECTION: How did you see God move in the events of this month? (If this is hard to see, ask Him to help you interpret the events).

11 Sh'vat | January – February

TRIBE	ALPHABET	NUMBER	CONSTELLATION
Asher	*TZADI*	11	Aquarius

Jacob + Zilpah = Asher

GENESIS 30:12-13 CJB | 12 Zilpah, Le'ah's slave-girl bore Ya'akov [Jacob] a second son; 13 and Le'ah said, "How happy I am! Women will say I am happy!" and called him Asher [happy].

The Blessing Of Jacob…

GENESIS 49:20 CJB | 20 "Asher's food is rich — he will provide food fit for a king.

The Blessing Of Moses…

DEUTERONOMY 33:24-25 CJB | 24 Of Asher he said: "May Asher be most blessed of sons; may he be the favorite among his brothers and bathe his feet in oil.
25 May your bolts be of iron and bronze and your strength last as long as you live.

Historical and biblical context. *Sh'vat* is known as a month of renewal in the agricultural cycle of Israel. The fifteenth day of *Sh'vat*, known as *Tu BiSh'vat* is celebrated as the "New Year for Trees," marking the period when the sap inside trees begins to increase, signifying a new agricultural season is about to begin. This day holds special significance because of its connection to the land and the promises of God's provision and sustenance for His people.

Sh'vat is also connected to Moses' final words to Israel before they entered the Promised Land. According to Deuteronomy 1:3, Moses taught the *Torah* to the Israelites on the first day of *Sh'vat* which connects his teaching and instruction to spiritual growth and preparation.

The tribe of Asher. The month of *Sh'vat* is traditionally linked to the tribe of Asher, one of the twelve sons of Jacob, and his name means "happy" or "blessed" (Genesis 30:13). Asher's territory was known for its fertile lands and abundance of olive oil (Deuteronomy 33:24), which corresponds rather nicely with the agricultural renewal that begins in *Sh'vat*. The tribe of Asher's association with prosperity and blessing reflects the idea of God's provision and care for His people, particularly in relation to the land.

According to Marty Solomon, the ties between the land and God's promises illustrate how Asher's blessing of fertility and prosperity symbolize the abundance that comes from living in alignment with God's purposes. *Sh'vat*, as a time of agricultural renewal, reminds us of the fruitfulness that comes from being rooted in God's Word and His promises.

The letter Tzadi. *Sh'vat* is associated with the Hebrew letter *Tzadi* ["righteous"] and symbolizes the larger concept of righteousness, as the word *Tzadik* means "righteous person." Scholars believe the shape of the letter can also represent a person in prayer or seeking justice.

According to Dr. Michael S. Heiser, the biblical theme of righteousness and justice is central to understanding God's covenant with His people. He notes that in the context of *Sh'vat*, the letter *Tzadi* symbolically invites believers to reflect on their personal growth in righteousness, especially as the natural world around them begins its renewal. The letter reminds us that our spiritual renewal and alignment with God's righteousness is essential preparation for new growth.

The number eleven. *Sh'vat,* as the eleventh month of the Hebrew calendar, is associated with the number eleven (11) and symbolizes disorder or incompletion, as it falls just short of the completeness represented by the number twelve (e.g., Israel's twelve tribes or divine government).

However, in the context of *Sh'vat*, this number also points to a time of transition and preparation, especially since it precedes the month of *Adar*, when *Purim* (a time of deliverance) is celebrated.

According to Marty Solomon, recognizing these times of preparation and waiting is crucial for spiritual growth. Thus, *Sh'vat* is a month for us to focus on planting seeds of righteousness that will bear future fruit.

The constellation Aquarius. *Sh'vat* is associated with the constellation of Aquarius [Heb. *D'li*] and is symbolized as the water-bearer. Water is a powerful biblical symbol, often embodying life, renewal, and the Spirit of God (Isaiah 44:3). In the context of *Sh'vat*, the water-bearer represents the outpouring of God's blessings and the renewal of life, both physically through the land and spiritually through union with God.

According to Dr. G. K. Beale, water, particularly in biblical eschatology, signifies life and the renewal of creation. For example, in Revelation 22, the river of life flows from the throne of God, renewing all things.

Sh'vat's link to Aquarius invites us to anticipate this time of renewal and to seek spiritual refreshment as we look forward to eternal renewal in Yeshua.

Spiritual focus of Sh'vat. For followers of Yeshua, the month of *Sh'vat* carries deep spiritual connections to renewal, growth, and preparation. The agricultural renewal that begins in *Sh'vat* mirrors the spiritual renewal that we are called to pursue as we align ourselves with God's purposes.

We set aside time to remember the fruitfulness that living in alignment with God's will produces, and to seek a deeper understanding of His righteousness and justice. It is a time for self-examination, prayer, and aligning one's life with God's standards.

Although we live in a constant state of preparation for what God will do, *Sh'vat* is an especially important time to intentionally prepare the soil of one's heart for the blessings and growth that God will bring in the coming season.

Although always available, this is the month to draw from the outpouring of God's Spirit and the refreshment that comes from the living water that flows through Yeshua.

> **JOHN 4:14 CJB** | [...] 14 but whoever drinks the water I [Yeshua] will give him will never be thirsty again! On the contrary, the water I give him will become a spring of water inside him, welling up into eternal life!"

Alignment in Sh'vat. The reason we process each month is to remain in alignment with God's rhythm of life. This means that we fearlessly examine both the good and the bad that happened each month to know where to invite God for healing, encouragement, direction, blessing, or repentance.

We believe that *unresolved grief is undelivered communication of an emotional nature.* When these communications (either positive or negative) are identified and expressed...*we experience emotional completion*. This enables us to keep our our hearts *clear* and *connected* as we practice alignment with God...instead of carrying our wounds and burdens into the next month.

Here's how we're going to use the Graphing Tool on the following pages:

STEP NO. 1: On the graph, start at the **BEGINNING OF MONTH** and continue to the **END OF MONTH**...

- Write down any events that happened, with positive events above the line and negative events below the line.
- Draw a line to represent the intensity of the event (the longer the line, the greater the intensity).
- Label each event with one of these emotional components:
  A = Apology • F = Forgive • S = Significant Emotional Statement

STEP NO. 2: Write out a **Significant Emotional Statement** for each event. This represents your emotional truth about how this event affected you. Some events can also have an **Apology** or a **Forgive** included in the statement and might be addressed to God, to another person, or even to yourself.

Reflect on the past month and write out (1) anything you need to apologize for, (2) anything you need to forgive, and (3) anything that describes your emotional truth. (Remember there is no judgment here...this is just for your heart to be clear, so be honest!)

STEP NO. 3: Write down anything that comes to your mind when you reflect on how God has shown up in these events.

In our monthly *Zoom Coaching* call, Inspired Life members will read their sentences and connections to their partner.

THE HEBREW MONTHS

END OF MONTH

STEP NO. 1

A = Apologies • F = Forgives • SES = Positive Significant Emotional Statements

Positive is above the line | **Negative** is below the line

BEGINNING OF MONTH

STEP NO. 2

A = Apologies

F = Forgives

SES = Positive Significant Emotional Statements

REFLECTION: How did you see God move in the events of this month? (If this is hard to see, ask Him to help you interpret the events).

STEP NO. 3

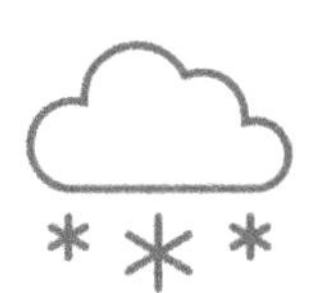

12 Adar | February – March

TRIBE	ALPHABET	NUMBER	CONSTELLATION
Naphtali	*KUF*	12	Pisces

Jacob + Bilhah = Naphtali

GENESIS 30:7-8 CJB | 7 Bilhah, Rachel's slave-girl conceived again and bore Ya'akov [Jacob] a second son. 8 Rachel said, "I have wrestled mightily with my sister and won," and called him Naftali [my wrestling].

The Blessing Of Jacob…

GENESIS 49:21 CJB | 21 Naftali [Naphtali] is a doe set free that bears beautiful fawns.

The Blessing Of Moses…

DEUTERONOMY 33:23 CJB | 23 Of Naftali he said: "You, Naftali, satisfied with favor and full of blessing from ADONAI, take possession of the sea and the south."

Historical and biblical context. The primary event associated with *Adar* is *Purim* which is celebrated on the 14th of *Adar* and commemorates the deliverance of the Jewish people from Haman's genocidal persecution as recorded in the book of Esther. This festival is joyfully celebrated with feasting and the giving of gifts (Esther 9:1-22).

The name *Adar* is derived from the Akkadian word *adaru*, meaning "strength" or "power." In this sense, the month reflects God's providential power to deliver His people from seemingly hopeless situations. For believers, this points to God's sovereignty and is demonstrated in the salvation that culminates in Yeshua's victory over sin and death (Colossians 2:15).

The tribe of Naphtali. The month of *Adar* is traditionally associated with the tribe of Naphtali, one of Jacob's twelve sons, and his name is described as "a doe set free that bears beautiful fawns" (Genesis 49:21). This description highlights themes of freedom and swiftness.

The tribe of Naphtali settled in the northwest region of Israel in an area that would later be associated with the ministry of Yeshua, particularly around the Sea of Galilee (Matthew 4:12-16).

According to Marty Solomon, freedom plays a significant role in biblical narratives, as illustrated by how often God delivers His people from oppression. Thus, the association of *Adar* with the tribe of Naphtali forms an important connection to the themes of deliverance and joy that define the month.

For followers of Yeshua, this reflects the freedom he offers us from spiritual bondage (John 8:36).

The letter Kuf. *Adar* is associated with the Hebrew letter *Kuf* ["holiness"] which visually resembles a person bowing in humility and represents holiness and the pursuit of God's ways. The letter is often associated with the concept of separating the holy from the profane which echoes the story of *Purim* when the Jews were called to maintain their spiritual identity and faithfulness to God even in the face of cultural assimilation and harsh persecution.

According to Dr. Michael S. Heiser, since holiness defined as being set apart for God's purposes, the association of *Adar* with *Kuf* reminds us to live lives of holiness while recognizing that deliverance comes from God's sovereign work and our faithfulness to Him (1 Peter 1:15-16).

The call to holiness in the face of adversity also mirrors the way Esther and Mordecai remained faithful to God despite living in exile.

The number twelve. *Adar,* as the twelfth month of the Hebrew calendar, is associated with the number twelve (12) which represents divine order and completeness (e.g., the twelve tribes of Israel; the twelve apostles of Yeshua, etc.) and points to spiritual fulfillment, particularly regarding God's promises in His overarching plan for redemption.

According to Dr. G. K. Beale, the Old Testament illustrates the theme of biblical fulfillment in the ultimate completion of God's redemptive plan through Yeshua. As the twelfth month, *Adar* signals the completion of the yearly cycle and invites believers to reflect on the fullness of God's deliverance...both in the historical events of *Purim* and in the final deliverance that comes through Yeshua.

The constellation Pisces. *Adar* is associated with the constellation Pisces [Heb. *Dagim*] meaning "fish." Fish are a common symbol in Scripture, representing abundance and provision (e.g., the multiplication of fish in Matthew 14:17-21). In the context of *Adar*, Pisces symbolizes the hidden abundance and provision of God, which can appear even in the most difficult and uncertain times.

According to Marty Solomon, fish, particularly in the New Testament, also illustrate discipleship. He notes that the calling of the disciples to be "fishers of men" (Matthew 4:19) connects the symbolism of Pisces with the theme of calling and mission. *Adar*, as the month of hidden deliverance and joy, encourages believers to trust in God's provision and to be active participants in His redemptive mission.

Spiritual focus of Adar. *Adar* is a time to reflect on the joy that comes from spiritual deliverance through Yeshua (John 15:11) and to embrace our freedom in him to speak words of truth and life. We are meant to discover and live out to the full calling that God has placed on our lives...even in difficult circumstances.

God uses this calling to invite us into a life set apart for Him in wholeness and holiness...to remain faithful to Him despite the pressures of the world...and to fully entrust ourselves to Him for deliverance. As we choose to rest in God's deliverance, His assurance becomes both our present reality and our future hope.

Alignment in Adar. The reason we process each month is to remain in alignment with God's rhythm of life. This means that we fearlessly examine both the good and the bad that happened each month to know where to invite God for healing, encouragement, direction, blessing, or repentance.

We believe that *unresolved grief is undelivered communication of an emotional nature.* When these communications (either positive or negative) are identified and expressed...*we experience emotional completion*. This enables us to keep our our hearts *clear* and *connected* as we practice alignment with God...instead of carrying our wounds and burdens into the next month.

Here's how we're going to use the Graphing Tool on the following pages:

STEP NO. 1: On the graph, start at the **BEGINNING OF MONTH** and continue to the **END OF MONTH**...

- Write down any events that happened, with positive events above the line and negative events below the line.
- Draw a line to represent the intensity of the event (the longer the line, the greater the intensity).
- Label each event with one of these emotional components:
  A = Apology • F = Forgive • S = Significant Emotional Statement

STEP NO. 2: Write out a **Significant Emotional Statement** for each event. This represents your emotional truth about how this event affected you. Some events can also have an **Apology** or a **Forgive** included in the statement and might be addressed to God, to another person, or even to yourself.

Reflect on the past month and write out (1) anything you need to apologize for, (2) anything you need to forgive, and (3) anything that describes your emotional truth. (Remember there is no judgment here...this is just for your heart to be clear, so be honest!)

STEP NO. 3: Write down anything that comes to your mind when you reflect on how God has shown up in these events.

In our monthly *Zoom Coaching* call, Inspired Life members will read their sentences and connections to their partner.

THE HEBREW MONTHS

END OF MONTH

STEP NO. 1

A = Apologies • F = Forgives • SES = Positive Significant Emotional Statements

Positive is above the line | **Negative** is below the line

BEGINNING OF MONTH

STEP NO. 2

A = Apologies

F = Forgives

SES = Positive Significant Emotional Statements

REFLECTION: How did you see God move in the events of this month? (If this is hard to see, ask Him to help you interpret the events).

STEP NO. 3

SPRING | **Nissan**

1 Nissan | March – April
2 Iyyar | April – May
3 Sivan | May – June

Spring [Heb. Aviv] is a time of new beginnings, renewal, and redemption. Agriculturally, it is the season of barley and wheat harvests and marks the start of Israel's agricultural cycle.

Spiritually, spring corresponds to the celebration of Peshach [Passover], which commemorates the Israelites' Exodus from Egypt (Exodus 12). This season is deeply tied to the theme of deliverance, as the Israelites were freed from slavery and began their journey toward the Promised Land.

According to Marty Solomon, spring is a time of spiritual awakening, when God brings His people out of bondage and sets them on a path of spiritual growth. The counting of the Omer also begins in spring, symbolizing the spiritual preparation for the giving of the Torah at Shavuot [Pentecost] in the next season.

Dr. G. K. Beale has noted the typological significance of the Passover lamb in Christian theology, where spring marks the crucifixion and resurrection of Yeshua...the ultimate fulfillment of Israel's deliverance. Therefore, the season of spring in the Hebrew calendar is a time of renewal, both agriculturally and spiritually, marking the beginning of God's redemptive work in history.

1 Nissan ["beginning of barley harvest] • **2 Iyyar** ["barley harvest"] • **3 Sivan** ["wheat harvest"]

SIDE NOTE: The Hebrew calendar originally began with the month of *Tishre*i, but when God established Passover, Israel entered into an annual cycle of redemption, and He commanded that *Nissan* be marked as the "head of the months." In fact, the first commandment given to the Hebrews as they prepared to leave Egypt was, "You are to begin your calendar with this month [*Nissan*]; it will be the first month of the year for you." (Exodus 12:2 CJB)

Consequently, the Hebrew years are still numbered from *Tishrei* (the month when we celebrate *Rosh Hashanah*) but the months are now numbered from *Nissan*. That is why the Jewish new year begins at the start of the seventh month.

01 Nissan | March - April

TRIBE	ALPHABET	NUMBER	CONSTELLATION
Judah	*HEI*	1	Aries

Jacob + Leah = Judah

GENESIS 29:34 CJB | 34 She [Le'ah] conceived yet again, had a son and said, "This time I will praise ADONAI"; therefore, she named him Y'hudah [praise]. Then she stopped having children.

The Blessing Of Jacob...

GENESIS 49:8-12 CJB | 8 "Y'hudah [Judah], your brothers will acknowledge you, your hand will be on the neck of your enemies, your father's sons will bow down before you. 9 Y'hudah is a lion's cub; my son, you stand over the prey. He crouches down and stretches like a lion; like a lioness, who dares to provoke him? 10 The scepter will not pass from Y'hudah, nor the ruler's staff from between his legs, until he comes to whom [obedience] belongs; and it is he whom the peoples will obey. 11 Tying his donkey to the vine, his donkey's colt to the choice grapevine, he washes his clothes in wine, his robes in the blood of grapes. 12 His eyes will be darker than wine, his teeth whiter than milk.

The Blessing Of Moses...

DEUTERONOMY 33:7 CJB | 7 Of Y'hudah [Judah] he said: "Hear, ADONAI, the cry of Y'hudah! Bring him into his people, let his own hands defend him; but you, help him against his enemies."

Historical and biblical context. The Hebrew month of *Nissan* is central to biblical history as the time when the Jews were liberated from slavery in Egypt. In Exodus 12, God commands His people to observe Passover on the 14th of *Nissan* which commemorates the pivotal moment when the Angel of Death "passed over" the homes of Hebrews marked with the blood of the lamb. This liberation became the defining moment of Israel's identity as God's chosen people and the foundation of their covenant relationship with Him.

For us, *Nissan* carries even greater significance as the month of Yeshua's death and resurrection. He was the ultimate Passover Lamb for all of humanity and his sacrifice delivers us from the power of sin and death.

According to Dr. Michael S. Heiser, the typological connections between the Old Testament sacrificial system and Yeshua emphasizes how *Nissan* serves as the backdrop for the fulfillment of God's redemptive plan in Yeshua.

> **1 CORINTHIANS 5:7 CJB** | 7 Get rid of the old hametz [leaven], so that you can be a new batch of dough, because in reality you are unleavened. For our Pesach [Passover] lamb, the Messiah, has been sacrificed.

The tribe of Judah. The month of *Nissan* is associated with the tribe of Judah, one of Jacob's twelve sons, and became the royal tribe from which King David, and ultimately Yeshua, the Messiah, descended. Genesis 49:8-10 describes Judah as the tribe destined for leadership, saying, "The scepter will not pass from Judah."

Judah both represents and includes the four letters of the *Havayah* [the four-letter Hebrew word for the name of the God]. Judah also embodies the path of selflessness [Heb. *bittul*]...the most vital ingredient of true leadership.

According to Marty Solomon, the tribe of Judah represents kingship, leadership, and ultimately the Messianic promise. The tribe's association with *Nissan* highlights both of these themes (redemption and kingship) which are central to Passover and the coming of the Messiah. It is rather fitting then, that as the first month, *Nissan* is linked to the tribe from which the eternal King

(Yeshua) would come, symbolizing his earthly and divine rulership.

The letter Hei. *Nissan* is associated with the Hebrew letter *Hei* ["the"] and represents the idea of "breath" or "revelation" as it symbolizes the divine presence or God's breath [Heb. *ruach*]. The letter *Hei* also appears in the sacred name of God (*YHWH*) and exemplifies His creative power.

According to Dr. G. K. Beale, God's presence and revelation in Scripture is often illustrated during key moments of deliverance and redemption that are directly tied to God revealing Himself to His people.

In the context of *Nissan*, the letter *Hei* reminds us of God's direct participation in human history, particularly in the redemption of Israel from Egypt and the revelation of His covenant at Sinai. For believers, this divine involvement finds its ultimate expression in the revelation of Yeshua as the Savior of the world, whose death and resurrection occurred during *Nissan*.

The number one. *Nissan*, as the first month of the Hebrew calendar, is associated with the number one (1) which symbolizes unity, beginnings, and primacy. It is the number that represents God's oneness and His uniquely sovereign role as Creator and Redeemer, "Hear, Isra'el! ADONAI our God, ADONAI is one" (Deuteronomy 6:4 CJB).

The number one in the context of *Nissan* signifies the beginning of the sacred year and highlights the foundational nature of the Exodus story in Israel's identity. For us, the significance of *Nissan* as the first month of the year parallels the idea that Yeshua's death and resurrection during this time marked the beginning of a new covenant and the inauguration of God's kingdom on earth (Hebrews 9:15).

As co-heirs to this new covenant, we are now a new creation and offered a new beginning through Yeshua.

The constellation Aries. *Nissan* is associated with the constellation of Aries [Heb. *Taleh*] which is represented as a ram or lamb. Aries is particularly fitting for *Nissan*, since the sacrificial lamb is central to the Passover story as (1) the key symbol of deliverance for the Israelites and (2) its blood was used for marking the doors of their homes, sparing them from the final plague of death.

The symbolism of the lamb is also represented in the person of Yeshua, "the Lamb of God" (John 1:29) whose sacrificial death brings salvation to the world. The constellation of Aries reinforces the idea of sacrifice and redemption, linking *Nissan* to the overarching biblical narrative of God's deliverance of His people, first through the Passover, and later through Yeshua's atoning death.

Spiritual focus of Nissan. The month of *Nissan* is a time of redemption, new beginnings, and divine revelation and represents a turning point in both Jewish and Christian history, when God's deliverance was manifested in powerful and tangible ways.

The deliverance of Israel during *Nissan* foreshadowed the sacrifice (and later reign of Yeshua) and directs our attention to whatever is competing with his lordship in our lives...to whatever we are prioritizing ahead of him...and to seeking our *shalom* ["well-being"; "wellness"; "good health"; "wholeness"] IN HIM.

As the first month, *Nissan* sets the spiritual tone for the rest of the year. The Exodus marked the beginning of Israel's national identity as a people redeemed by God, and for Christians, *Nissan* ushers in the new creation that comes through the resurrection of Yeshua.

Nissan is also a time to reflect on the power of God's deliverance, the hope of new beginnings, and the fulfillment of His promises, making it a foundational month for both the Jewish and Messianic communities.

Alignment in Nissan. The reason we process each month is to remain in alignment with God's rhythm of life. This means that we fearlessly examine both the good and the bad that happened each month to know where to invite God for healing, encouragement, direction, blessing, or repentance.

We believe that *unresolved grief is undelivered communication of an emotional nature.* When these communications (either positive or negative) are identified and expressed...*we experience emotional completion*. This enables us to keep our our hearts *clear* and *connected* as we practice alignment with God...instead of carrying our wounds and burdens into the next month.

Here's how we're going to use the Graphing Tool on the following pages:

STEP NO. 1: On the graph, start at the **BEGINNING OF MONTH** and continue to the **END OF MONTH**...

- Write down any events that happened, with positive events above the line and negative events below the line.
- Draw a line to represent the intensity of the event (the longer the line, the greater the intensity).
- Label each event with one of these emotional components:
  A = Apology • F = Forgive • S = Significant Emotional Statement

STEP NO. 2: Write out a **Significant Emotional Statement** for each event. This represents your emotional truth about how this event affected you. Some events can also have an **Apology** or a **Forgive** included in the statement and might be addressed to God, to another person, or even to yourself.

Reflect on the past month and write out (1) anything you need to apologize for, (2) anything you need to forgive, and (3) anything that describes your emotional truth. (Remember there is no judgment here...this is just for your heart to be clear, so be honest!)

STEP NO. 3: Write down anything that comes to your mind when you reflect on how God has shown up in these events.

In our monthly *Zoom Coaching* call, Inspired Life members will read their sentences and connections to their partner.

THE HEBREW MONTHS

END OF MONTH

STEP NO. 1

A = Apologies • F = Forgives • SES = Positive Significant Emotional Statements

Positive is above the line | **Negative** is below the line

BEGINNING OF MONTH

STEP NO. 2

A = Apologies

F = Forgives

SES = Positive Significant Emotional Statements

REFLECTION: How did you see God move in the events of this month? (If this is hard to see, ask Him to help you interpret the events).

STEP NO. 3

02 Iyyar | April – May

TRIBE	ALPHABET	NUMBER	CONSTELLATION
Issachar	*VAV*	2	Taurus

Jacob + Leah = Issachar

GENESIS 30:17-18 CJB | 17 God listened to Le'ah, and she conceived and bore Ya'akov [Jacob] a fifth son. 18 Le'ah said, "God has given me my hire, because I gave my slave-girl to my husband." So, she called him Yissakhar [hire, reward].

The Blessing Of Jacob...

GENESIS 49:14-15 CJB | 14 "Yissakhar [Issachar] is a strong donkey lying down in the sheep sheds. 15 On seeing how good is settled life and how pleasant the country, he will bend his back to the burden and submit to forced labor.

The Blessing Of Moses...

DEUTERONOMY 33:18-19 CJB | 18 Of Z'vulun [Zebulun] he said: "Rejoice, Z'vulun, as you go forth, and you, Yissakhar, in your tents. 19 They will summon peoples to the mountain and there offer righteous sacrifices; for they will draw from the abundance of the seas and from the hidden treasures of the sand."

Historical and biblical context. The Hebrew month of *Iyyar*, referred to as *Ziv* in some biblical texts (1 Kings 6:1), is significant in Jewish history (and our own spiritual reflection) as it serves as a bridge between the freedom of Passover [*Pesach*] in the preceding month of *Nissan* and the revelation of the *Torah* at

Pentecost [*Shavuot*] in the following month of *Sivan*. *Iyyar* is also marked by the counting of the *Omer*, a period of anticipation and preparation between *Pesach* [Passover] and *Shavuot* [Pentecost].

This is why the Hebrew month of *Iyyar* represents a month of transition. For example, after their deliverance from Egypt in *Nissan*, the Israelites traveled in the wilderness during *Iyyar*. During this time, they experienced God's provision in the form of manna (Exodus 16) and water from the rock (Exodus 17:1-7). Thus, *Iyyar* was a period of healing, preparation, and provision as the people journeyed to Mount Sinai to receive the *Torah*.

According to Marty Solomon, the themes of waiting and growth during the month of *Iyyar* are illustrated by the Israelites learning to trust in God's daily provision while they moved from the celebration of freedom [*Pesach*] toward the revelation of God's covenant at Mount Sinai [*Shavuot]*. This waiting period also aligns with the counting of the *Omer*, a 49-day process to help the Hebrews spiritually prepare to receive God's Word.

One of the names associated with *Iyyar* is the *Chodesh Ziv* ["Month of Healing"] because it was when God revealed Himself as *Yahweh-Rapha* ["the Lord who heals"] (Exodus 15:26). After the waters at Marah were purified, God promised Israel that they could avoid being afflicted with the diseases of Egypt by remaining obedient to Him...for He is their healer. Thus, *Iyyar* is a time of physical and spiritual healing, in which the entire community reflected on God's ability to make them whole.

According to Dr. Michael S. Heiser, the implications of God's physical and spiritual provision are exemplified in the relationship between healing and divine deliverance. For example, the healing waters at Marah represented God's *restorative work*, while the manna and quail in the wilderness reminded Israel of God's *continued care*.

The tribe of Issachar. The month of *Iyyar* is associated with the tribe of Issachar, one of Jacob's twelve sons, and is described in 1 Chronicles 12:33 CJB as a tribe that "understood the times" and knew "what Israel ought to do." This suggests that Issachar possessed a unique ability to discern the seasons and align with God's timing.

According to Marty Solomon, the importance of discernment in spiritual journeys was especially evident during the transitional times of *Iyyar*. The tribe of Issachar, with its insight into the times and seasons, encourages us to use this month to seek God's guidance and to align our lives with His will. *Iyyar* is also a month of preparation, and like Issachar, we are called to understand the times and make decisions in line with God's purposes.

The letter Vav. *Iyyar* is associated with the Hebrew letter *Vav* ["and"] and is used as a conjunction. In the Hebrew language it links words, phrases, and ideas, symbolizing both connection and continuity. In the context of *Iyyar*, this represents the connection between *Pesach*/Passover (the celebration of freedom) and *Shavuot*/Pentecost (the giving of the *Torah*), as well as the relationship between heaven and earth.

According to Dr. G. K. Beale, the correlation between earthly events and divine purposes in Scripture is beautifully illustrated during *Iyyar*, as the letter *Vav* reminds us of our connection to God and to each other, emphasizing the importance of unity and cohesion within the Messianic community. Spiritually, *Iyyar* is a time to reflect on the relationship between our physical needs and spiritual growth, recognizing that *both come from God's provision*.

The number two. *Iyyar*, as the second month of the Hebrew calendar, is associated with the number two (2) and represents duality, partnership, and witness. For example, in the *Torah*, legal matters often required the testimony of two witnesses (Deuteronomy 19:15). In the context of *Iyyar*, the number two signifies the partnership between God and Israel as they journeyed through the wilderness and learned to rely on Him as their guide and provider.

According to Dr. Michael S. Heiser, the number two can also represent the tension between earthly and heavenly realms, as evidenced in biblical cosmology (i.e., the biblical account of the universe and its laws).

During *Iyyar*, this tension was especially evident when the Israelites, freed from physical bondage in Egypt, were preparing for God's revelation at Mount Sinai. The duality of *Iyyar* reminds us that both physical and spiritual provision come from God, and we must navigate these realities with trust and faith.

The constellation Taurus. *Iyyar* is associated with the constellation of Taurus [Heb. *Shor*] which is represented as a bull. In the ancient world, bulls symbolized strength, stamina, and productivity. The bull embodies the strength and endurance required to journey through the wilderness in order to reach Mount Sinai.

In Scripture, the bull is often associated with sacrificial offerings (Leviticus 4:3). During *Iyyar*, while the Israelites journeyed through the wilderness, God taught them about sacrifice and obedience. According to Marty Solomon, these wilderness travels represented a testing of God's people, in much the same way that the bull symbolized both strength and sacrifice. Spiritually, the bull inspires us to persevere and to trust in God's provision even in challenging times.

Spiritual focus of Iyyar. The month of *Iyyar* is a time of transition, healing, and preparation as the Messianic community moves from the redemption of *Pesach*/Passover to the revelation of the *Torah* at *Shavuot*/Pentecost. It offers believers a time to reflect on God's ongoing provision, healing, and guidance.

Iyyar is often called the "Month of Healing" because it marks the time when God healed and provided for the Israelites as they traveled through the wilderness. For this reason, believers are encouraged to seek both physical and spiritual healing during this time, trusting in God to restore what is broken and provide for their needs.

Since *Iyyar* falls during the counting of the *Omer*, a time of anticipation and spiritual refinement, believers are also encouraged to prepare their hearts for deeper revelation and understanding, much like the Israelites prepared for the giving of the *Torah* at Mount Sinai.

Alignment in Iyyar. The reason we process each month is to remain in alignment with God's rhythm of life. This means that we fearlessly examine both the good and the bad that happened each month to know where to invite God for healing, encouragement, direction, blessing, or repentance.

We believe that *unresolved grief is undelivered communication of an emotional nature.* When these communications (either positive or negative) are identified and expressed...*we experience emotional completion*. This enables us to keep our our hearts *clear* and *connected* as we practice alignment with God...instead of carrying our wounds and burdens into the next month.

Here's how we're going to use the Graphing Tool on the following pages:

STEP NO. 1: On the graph, start at the **BEGINNING OF MONTH** and continue to the **END OF MONTH**...

- Write down any events that happened, with positive events above the line and negative events below the line.
- Draw a line to represent the intensity of the event (the longer the line, the greater the intensity).
- Label each event with one of these emotional components:
  A = Apology • F = Forgive • S = Significant Emotional Statement

STEP NO. 2: Write out a **Significant Emotional Statement** for each event. This represents your emotional truth about how this event affected you. Some events can also have an **Apology** or a **Forgive** included in the statement and might be addressed to God, to another person, or even to yourself.

Reflect on the past month and write out (1) anything you need to apologize for, (2) anything you need to forgive, and (3) anything that describes your emotional truth. (Remember there is no judgment here...this is just for your heart to be clear, so be honest!)

STEP NO. 3: Write down anything that comes to your mind when you reflect on how God has shown up in these events.

In our monthly *Zoom Coaching* call, Inspired Life members will read their sentences and connections to their partner.

THE HEBREW MONTHS

END OF MONTH

STEP NO. 1

A = Apologies • F = Forgives • SES = Positive Significant Emotional Statements

Positive is above the line | **Negative** is below the line

BEGINNING OF MONTH

STEP NO. 2

A = Apologies

F = Forgives

SES = Positive Significant Emotional Statements

REFLECTION: How did you see God move in the events of this month? (If this is hard to see, ask Him to help you interpret the events).

STEP NO. 3

03 Sivan | May – June

TRIBE	ALPHABET	NUMBER	CONSTELLATION
Zebulun	*ZAYIN*	3	Gemini

Jacob + Leah = Zebulun

GENESIS 30:19-20 CJB | 19 Le'ah conceived again and bore a sixth son to
Ya'akov [Jacob]. 20 Le'ah said, "God has given me a wonderful gift. Now at
last my husband will live with me, since I have borne him six sons." And she
called him Z'vulun [living together].

The Blessing Of Jacob...

GENESIS 49:13 CJB | 13 "Z'vulun [Zebulun] will live at the seashore, with ships anchoring along his coast and his border at Tzidon [Sidon].

The Blessing Of Moses...

DEUTERONOMY 33:18-19 CJB | 18 Of Z'vulun he said: "Rejoice, Z'vulun, as you go
forth, and you, Yissakhar [Issachar], in your tents. 19 They will summon
peoples to the mountain and there offer righteous sacrifices; for they will draw
from the abundance of the seas and from the hidden treasures of the sand."

Historical and biblical context. Zebulun later received the land between the Mediterranean Sea and Sea of Galilee and will assume possession of the land extending to the sea in the future Millennial Kingdom (Ezekiel 48:1-8, 23-27). However, this prophecy does not yet appear to have been fulfilled since it likely concerns the Millennium.

The Hebrew month of *Sivan* holds deep historical and spiritual significance in Scripture, most notably as the month of *Shavuot* ["Feast of Weeks"], which celebrates the giving of the *Torah* at Mount Sinai. This event marked a pivotal moment in Israel's history when the covenant between God and Israel was formally established through the *Torah*.

Consequently, the most significant event in *Sivan* is the celebration of *Shavuot* which takes place on the 6th of *Sivan*. This festival is considered the consummation of the Exodus...when God gave the *Torah* to the Israelites at Mount Sinai (Exodus 19-20)...and when their physical deliverance from Egypt in *Nissan* was followed by their spiritual deliverance through the revelation of God's laws.

According to Marty Solomon, the giving of the *Torah* formed the foundation of Israel's national identity. It was the moment when God formalized His covenant with Israel and instructed them how to live in relationship with Him and with one another. Thus, *Sivan* is a time of revelation and covenantal responsibility that reminds us of the importance of aligning our lives with God's word.

According Dr. Michael S. Heiser, the significance of the Mount Sinai revelation was fully revealed in the giving of the *Torah* during *Sivan* as it marked a key moment of divine communication when God made His will directly known to humanity and laid the foundation for Israel's understanding of justice, worship, and communal life.

The tribe of Zebulun. The month of *Sivan* is associated with the tribe of Zebulun, one of Jacob's twelve sons, and is traditionally linked with commerce and trade. In Genesis 49:13, Jacob's blessing declares that the tribe will "live at the seashore," signifying its role in maritime trade and commerce.

The tribe of Zebulun was also known for its close partnership with the tribe of Issachar, with Zebulun's commercial ventures financially supporting Issachar's study of *Torah*.

According to Marty Solomon, Zebulun represents the balance between the material and the spiritual...with the tribe's commercial prosperity understood as a material support for the spiritual pursuits of others, particularly the *Torah* scholars of Issachar.

In the context of *Sivan*, this reflects the spiritual principle that our material resources and blessings are given by God to support the pursuit of His truth, wisdom, and purpose. Thus, the month of *Sivan* is an opportunity to reflect on how our resources can be used in service of God's kingdom and the well-being of others.

The letter Zayin. *Sivan* is associated with the Hebrew letter *Zayin* ["weapon"] and represents either a weapon or more specifically, a sword. In biblical terms, a sword exemplified both physical and spiritual warfare. For example, in Ephesians 6:17 CJB, we are encouraged to wield "the sword given by the Spirit, that is, the Word of God" to wage war. The association of the letter *Zayin* with the month of *Sivan* highlights the spiritual battle involved in receiving and living according to God's law.

According to Marty Solomon, the *Torah* is a "weapon" against chaos, sin, and injustice. It is not merely a set of rules but a tool for shaping a just society and guiding God's people through life's challenges. He views *Sivan* as a time for spiritual reflection on how God's word equips us to confront the challenges of life, whether they be spiritual, personal, or communal.

According to Dr. G. K. Beale, the letter *Zayin* symbolizes spiritual warfare and highlights the need for faithfulness in order to be victorious. For example, when God gave Israel the *Torah* at Mount Sinai and called them to live as a holy people surrounded by pagan nations...*it was a spiritual commitment* to a battle that God was preparing them to win. Likewise, the letter *Zayin* reminds us to arm ourselves with God's word as we strive to remain faithful to His promises.

The number three. *Sivan*, as the third month of the Hebrew calendar, is associated with the number three (3) which represents completeness and stability and often signifies the establishment of something solid (e.g., the three patriarchs, Abraham, Isaac, and Jacob; the three pilgrimage festivals, *Pesach*, *Shavuot*, and *Sukkot*).

In the context of *Sivan*, the number three reflects the completion of the journey from the Exodus (*Nissan*) to the giving of the *Torah* (*Sivan*). It symbolizes the moment when Israel, having been delivered from Egypt and purified in the wilderness, was spiritually prepared to receive divine revelation and enter a covenantal relationship with God.

According to Dr. Michael S. Heiser, the number three is often associated with divine action and the fulfillment of God's promises. In *Sivan*, we see the fulfillment of God's promise to lead Israel out of slavery and into a new life governed by His law. Spiritually, this number encourages us to reflect on the importance of establishing solid foundations in our walk with God, particularly through studying and obeying His word.

The constellation Gemini. *Sivan* is associated with the constellation of Gemini [Heb. *Te'omim*] which means "The Twins." In Hebrew tradition, twins often symbolized unity and complementary opposites. While the exact biblical significance of constellations is not heavily emphasized here, Gemini's association with duality reflects the larger idea of balance and harmony.

In the spiritual context of *Sivan*, Gemini symbolizes the dual aspect of the physical (earthly) and spiritual (heavenly) realms. Receiving the *Torah* at Mount Sinai was not just a spiritual event, but also an earthly covenant that governed the daily lives of God's people.

According to Marty Solomon, the *Torah* was the means through which God intended Israel to unite the physical and the spiritual in order to convert common, everyday actions into a reflection of divine principles. Gemini's symbolism serves as a reminder that spiritual truths must be lived out in the practical, everyday world.

According to Dr. G. K. Beale, the concept of twins, or complementary pairs, also reflects the relationship between God and Israel. Just as twins are bound together, the giving of the *Torah* binds God and Israel into a covenantal relationship. Thus, the constellation of Gemini symbolizes the unity and partnership between God and His people as they walk in obedience to wherever He leads them.

Spiritual focus of Sivan. The month of *Sivan* is a time of revelation, commitment, and covenant, when Israel stepped into its role as a holy nation with a clear understanding of its purpose.

Sivan is also a time to reflect on the gift of the *Torah* and the responsibility that comes with it. Though sobering, this encourages us to live holistic lives that integrate our material blessings with spiritual devotion.

The word of God serves as both guide and defense against sin and injustice, empowering us to successfully wage spiritual warfare and to attain ever-increasing maturity as we live our lives with whole-hearted devotion to God and His word.

Alignment in Sivan. The reason we process each month is to remain in alignment with God's rhythm of life. This means that we fearlessly examine both the good and the bad that happened each month to know where to invite God for healing, encouragement, direction, blessing, or repentance.

We believe that *unresolved grief is undelivered communication of an emotional nature.* When these communications (either positive or negative) are identified and expressed...*we experience emotional completion*. This enables us to keep our our hearts *clear* and *connected* as we practice alignment with God...instead of carrying our wounds and burdens into the next month.

Here's how we're going to use the Graphing Tool on the following pages:

STEP NO. 1: On the graph, start at the **BEGINNING OF MONTH** and continue to the **END OF MONTH**...

- Write down any events that happened, with positive events above the line and negative events below the line.
- Draw a line to represent the intensity of the event (the longer the line, the greater the intensity).
- Label each event with one of these emotional components:
  A = Apology • F = Forgive • S = Significant Emotional Statement

STEP NO. 2: Write out a **Significant Emotional Statement** for each event. This represents your emotional truth about how this event affected you. Some events can also have an **Apology** or a **Forgive** included in the statement and might be addressed to God, to another person, or even to yourself.

Reflect on the past month and write out (1) anything you need to apologize for, (2) anything you need to forgive, and (3) anything that describes your emotional truth. (Remember there is no judgment here...this is just for your heart to be clear, so be honest!)

STEP NO. 3: Write down anything that comes to your mind when you reflect on how God has shown up in these events.

In our monthly *Zoom Coaching* call, Inspired Life members will read their sentences and connections to their partner.

THE HEBREW MONTHS

END OF MONTH

STEP NO. 1

A = Apologies • F = Forgives • SES = Positive Significant Emotional Statements

Positive is above the line | **Negative** is below the line

BEGINNING OF MONTH

STEP NO. 2

A = Apologies

F = Forgives

SES = Positive Significant Emotional Statements

REFLECTION: How did you see God move in the events of this month? (If this is hard to see, ask Him to help you interpret the events).

STEP NO. 3

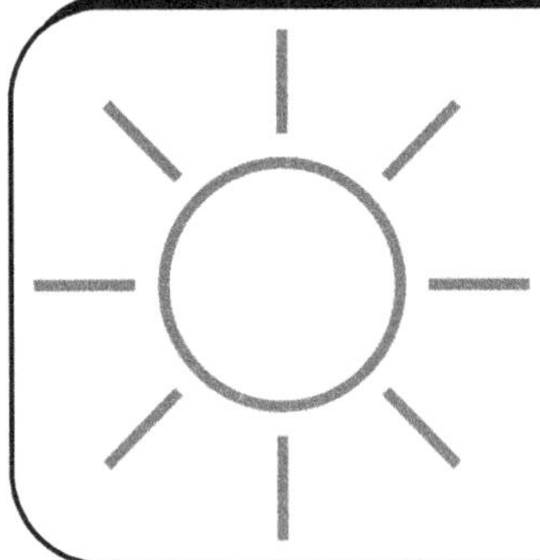

SUMMER | **Tammuz**

4 Tammuz | June – July
5 Av | July – August
6 Elul | August – September

Summer [Kayitz] is a time of harvest but also heat and a variety of other challenges. Agriculturally, it is when fruits like grapes, figs, and olives are harvested, signaling abundance...but it also requires hard work and endurance, as the intense heat of the season can be taxing on both crops and labor.

Spiritually, summer is marked by a period of mourning and reflection due to the historical tragedies associated with the season. The most notable event(s) being the destruction of both the First and Second Temples on the 9th of Av (Tisha B'Av).

Marty Solomon has observed that summer symbolizes a time of spiritual testing, when our faith is refined through adversity.

According to Dr. Michael S. Heiser, these themes of judgment and restoration are evidenced in summer's historical connection to Israel's greatest losses...which point to times of grief as well as the hope for redemption.

While summer represents harvest, it is also a period of recognizing the consequences of spiritual disobedience and the importance of repentance.

4 Tammuz ["harvesting"] • **5 Av** ["grapes, figs, and olives are ripe"] • **6 Elul** ["vintage begins"]

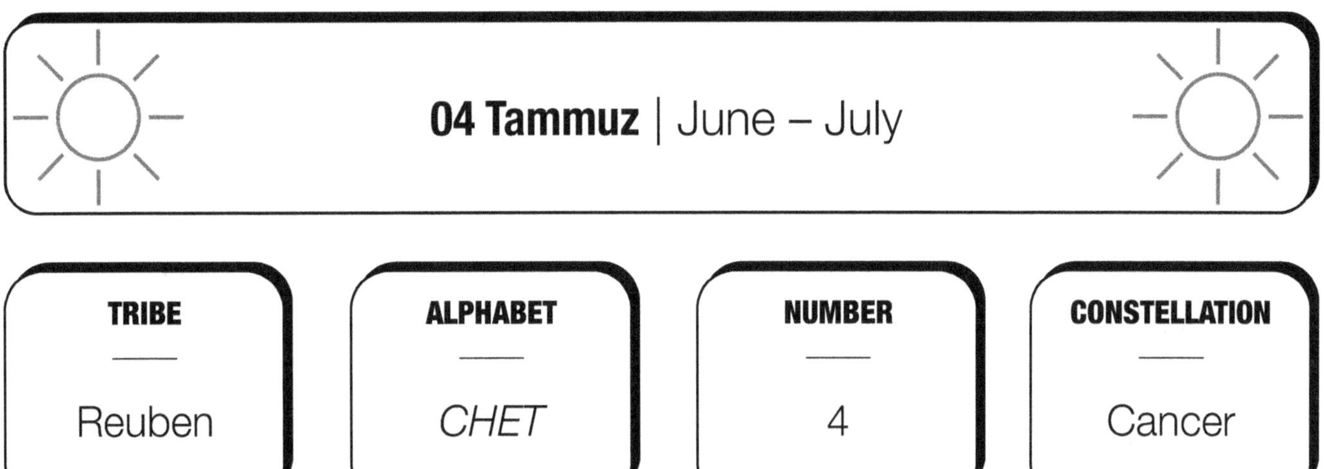

Jacob + Leah = Reuben

GENESIS 29:32 CJB | [32] Le'ah conceived and gave birth to a son, whom she named Re'uven [see, a son!], for she said, "It is because ADONAI has seen how humiliated I have been, but now my husband will love me."

The Blessing Of Jacob...

GENESIS 49:3-4 CJB | [3] "Re'uven [Reuben], you are my firstborn, my strength,
the first fruits of my manhood. [4] Though superior in vigor and power you are
unstable as water, so your superiority will end, because you climbed into your
father's bed and defiled it — he climbed onto my concubine's couch!

The Blessing Of Moses...

DEUTERONOMY 33:6 CJB | [6] "Let Re'uven live and not die out, even though his numbers grow few." (cf. Numbers 1:21; 2:11)

Historical and biblical context. The Hebrew month of *Tammuz* is historically linked to tragic events in the national life of Israel. The most significant of these events occurred on the 17th of *Tammuz* when the Babylonians breached the walls of Jerusalem and destroyed the First Temple (2 Kings 25:3-4, 8-9; Jeremiah 39:2, 8 CJB).

This day also marks the beginning of the "Three Weeks of Mourning" which culminates in *Tisha B'Av* (9th of *Av*), the day commemorating the destruction of both the First and Second Temples.

According to Marty Solomon, the events of *Tammuz* reflect the tragedy of spiritual failure and rebellion. Historically, *Tammuz* exemplifies moments in the national life of Israel when they failed to trust God and experienced His judgment. For example, upon witnessing Israel's worship of the golden calf Moses broke the tablets of the Law, with some sources suggesting that this likely occurred during *Tammuz* (Exodus 32). This episode illustrated Israel's abandonment of their covenant with God shortly after receiving the *Torah*.

Spiritually, *Tammuz* is a time of self-examination and repentance. It reminds believers of the dangers of idolatry and disobedience and calls upon us to reflect on our spiritual commitment to God.

According to Dr. Michael S. Heiser, the biblical concept of judgment is often intertwined with moments of spiritual failure and restoration. *Tammuz*, as a designated month of judgment, points to the consequences of abandoning God, the necessity of repentance, and our deep need to find refuge in His love.

The tribe of Reuben. The month of *Tammuz* is associated with the tribe of Reuben, one of Jacob's twelve sons. Reuben's life was marked by impulsiveness and regret, as evidenced when he dishonored his father by sleeping with Bilhah, Jacob's concubine (Genesis 35:22). This single impetuous act cost him his birthright (Genesis 49:4) which was later divided between Joseph's sons, Manasseh and Ephraim.

According to Marty Solomon, Reuben's actions represent a failure of self-control and a lack of personal responsibility...characteristics that resonate with the themes of *Tammuz*. Reuben's choices illustrate the dangers of impulsive acts and the lasting consequences of spiritual failure. *Tammuz*, much like Reuben's narrative, is a time to reflect (without self-shaming) on the consequences of one's actions and the importance of aligning one's life with God's word.

According to Dr. G. K. Beale, Reuben's failure does not signify permanent rejection but rather *reminds us of our need for restoration*. Like the nation of Israel in *Tammuz*, Reuben's story reassures us that while failure has very real consequences, *God's grace always leaves room for repentance*.

The letter Chet. *Tammuz* is associated with the Hebrew letter *Chet* ["separate"] which means life or boundary. In biblical terms, *Chet* signifies the boundary between life and death, or between holiness and sin. The form of the letter suggests an enclosure or protective wall which symbolizes the boundary that God establishes for His people through His commandments.

The association of the letter *Chet* with *Tammuz* reminds believers to stay within the loving protection of God's boundaries. Marty Solomon underscores this connection by noting that God's commandments are designed to preserve life and create order. When Israel crossed these boundaries (e.g., the idolatry of the golden calf) it led to death and destruction.

Thus, when the walls of Jerusalem were breached during *Tammuz*, it could be understood as both a literal and symbolic violation of God's protective boundaries.

According to Dr. Michael S. Heiser, boundaries in Scripture are never arbitrary but instead, reflect God's order and design for creation. *Tammuz*, marked by the breach of Jerusalem's walls, becomes a powerful reminder that while crossing God's boundaries leads to judgment...within those boundaries lies the fullness of life.

The number four. *Tammuz*, as the fourth month of the Hebrew calendar, is associated with the number four (4) which represents creation and the earthly realm and is also connected to the four cardinal directions and the four seasons, denoting completeness in the created world.

In the context of *Tammuz*, the number four represents the earthly consequences of spiritual actions. When boundaries are broken (e.g., the breach of Jerusalem's walls) it manifests in both physical and spiritual destruction.

The number four emphasizes this interconnectedness between the spiritual and the physical, highlighting the reality that spiritual disobedience produces real-world effects.

According to Dr. G. K. Beale, biblical numbers possess both theological and practical significance. For instance, the number four in *Tammuz* reminds us that our choices have both spiritual and material consequences that impact our life on earth.

The constellation Cancer. *Tammuz* is associated with the constellation of Cancer [Heb. *Sartan*] and is traditionally represented as a crab. In ancient Hebrew thought, Cancer was sometimes seen as representing a protective shell or the need for guarding and defense.

In the spiritual context of *Tammuz*, Cancer symbolizes the need for protection and watchfulness, particularly in times of spiritual crisis. Just as a crab relies on a hard shell to protect its vulnerable body, believers are reminded to guard their hearts and minds, especially during periods of temptation or trial.

> **PROVERBS 4:23 CJB** | [23] Above everything else, guard your heart; for it is the source of life's consequences.

During *Tammuz*, the walls of Jerusalem being breached remind believers that maintaining our spiritual defenses and remaining faithful to God's word is essential for our protection.

Marty Solomon and Dr. Michael S. Heiser have both highlighted the need for spiritual vigilance while noting that the image of Cancer's protective shell serves as an excellent metaphor for the spiritual boundaries God establishes through His law.

Tammuz challenges us to reflect on how well we are guarding our hearts and where we are vulnerable to "breaches" in our relationship with God.

Spiritual focus of Tammuz. The month of *Tammuz* is a time of tragedy, reflection, and spiritual testing, marked by historical events that resulted from Israel's disobedience and idolatry. *Tammuz* is a time to remember the consequences of crossing spiritual boundaries and to re-commit to restoring one's relationship with God through repentance and whole-heartedness.

This month is a period of sober reflection on the cost of rebellion against God, but also an opportunity for the refreshment and renewal that comes from repentance. We are called to examine our lives, restore our union with God, and rebuild our spiritual defenses with greater devotion and vigilance.

Alignment in Tammuz. The reason we process each month is to remain in alignment with God's rhythm of life. This means that we fearlessly examine both the good and the bad that happened each month to know where to invite God for healing, encouragement, direction, blessing, or repentance.

We believe that *unresolved grief is undelivered communication of an emotional nature.* When these communications (either positive or negative) are identified and expressed...*we experience emotional completion*. This enables us to keep our our hearts *clear* and *connected* as we practice alignment with God...instead of carrying our wounds and burdens into the next month.

Here's how we're going to use the Graphing Tool on the following pages:

STEP NO. 1: On the graph, start at the **BEGINNING OF MONTH** and continue to the **END OF MONTH**...

- Write down any events that happened, with positive events above the line and negative events below the line.
- Draw a line to represent the intensity of the event (the longer the line, the greater the intensity).
- Label each event with one of these emotional components:
  A = Apology • F = Forgive • S = Significant Emotional Statement

STEP NO. 2: Write out a **Significant Emotional Statement** for each event. This represents your emotional truth about how this event affected you. Some events can also have an **Apology** or a **Forgive** included in the statement and might be addressed to God, to another person, or even to yourself.

Reflect on the past month and write out (1) anything you need to apologize for, (2) anything you need to forgive, and (3) anything that describes your emotional truth. (Remember there is no judgment here...this is just for your heart to be clear, so be honest!)

STEP NO. 3: Write down anything that comes to your mind when you reflect on how God has shown up in these events.

In our monthly *Zoom Coaching* call, Inspired Life members will read their sentences and connections to their partner.

THE HEBREW MONTHS

END OF MONTH

STEP NO. 1

A = Apologies • F = Forgives • SES = Positive Significant Emotional Statements

Positive is above the line | **Negative** is below the line

BEGINNING OF MONTH

STEP NO. 2

A = Apologies

F = Forgives

SES = Positive Significant Emotional Statements

REFLECTION: How did you see God move in the events of this month? (If this is hard to see, ask Him to help you interpret the events).

STEP NO. 3

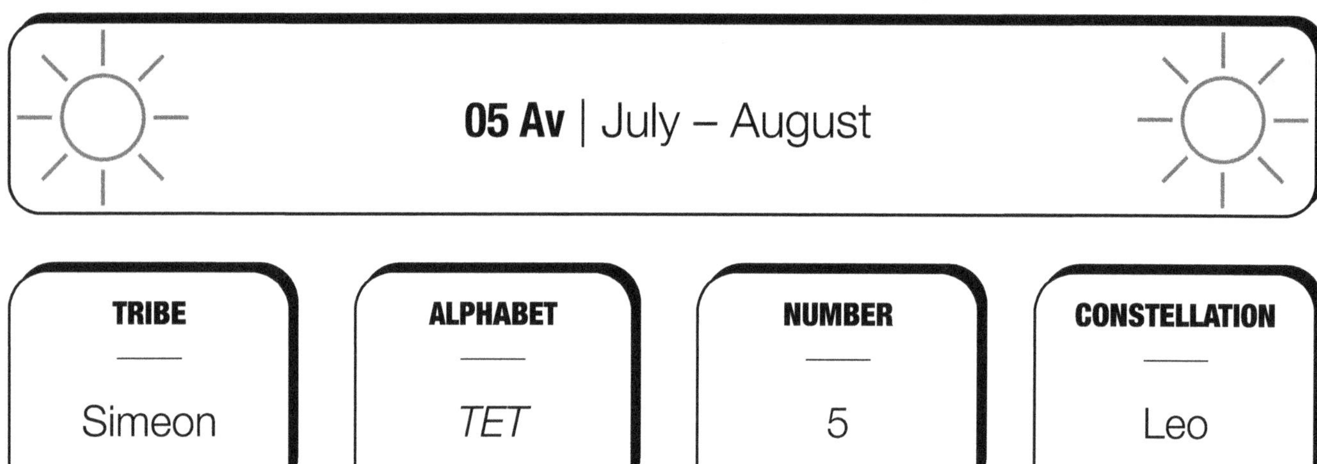

Jacob + Leah = Simeon

> **GENESIS 29:33 CJB** | [33] She [Le'ah] conceived again, gave birth to a son and said, "It is because ADONAI has heard that I am unloved; therefore, he has given me this son also." So, she named him Shim'on [hearing].

The Blessing Of Jacob...

> **GENESIS 49:5-7 CJB** | [5] "Shim'on [Simeon] and Levi are brothers, related by weapons of violence. [6] Let me not enter their council, let my honor not be connected with their people; for in their anger, they killed men, and at their whim they maimed cattle. [7] Cursed be their anger, for it has been fierce; their fury, for it has been cruel. I will divide them in Ya'akov [Jacob] and scatter them in Isra'el.

The Blessing Of Moses...

Simeon is the only one of the twelve tribes *not* blessed by Moses. The reason for this "omission" is that the tribe of Simeon was absorbed into Judah.

> **JOSHUA 19:1 CJB** | [1] The second lot came out for Shim'on [Simeon], for the tribe of the descendants of Shim'on according to their families. Their inheritance was inside the inheritance of the descendants of Y'hudah [Judah].

Historical and biblical context. The Hebrew month of *Av* is traditionally one of the most somber months due to several historical tragedies that occurred during this time. For instance, the 9th of *Av* [*Tisha B'Av*] is known as the saddest day on the Hebrew calendar as it marks the destruction of both the First Temple by the Babylonians (586 BC) and the Second Temple by the Romans (70 AD).

Other tragedies associated with this day include: the razing of Jerusalem by the Romans (c.136 AD), the expulsion of Jews from England (1290), the expulsion of Jews from Spain (1492), and the outbreak of World War I (1914).

According to Marty Solomon, *Tisha B'Av* illustrates the consequences of covenantal disobedience and spiritual decline, as demonstrated by Israel's failure to live up to its calling as a holy kingdom of priests.

Dr. Michael S. Heiser also notes that biblical judgment is closely entwined with covenant unfaithfulness. Thus, he views the month of *Av* a reflection of Israel's national failure. The destruction of the Temple, which symbolized God's presence among His people, represented a severe break in the relationship between God and Israel.

Although the month of *Av* is characterized by sorrow, it also precedes a time of consolation and hope. After *Tisha B'Av*, the Jewish calendar begins the "Seven Weeks of Consolation" and culminates in *Rosh Hashanah* [Jewish New Year]. This period is marked by prophetic readings of comfort to remind the people that God's mercy and restoration follow judgment. Marty Solomon has highlighted how God's story of redemption runs through these difficult times to demonstrate that destruction is not the end...*but rather a part of the larger narrative of renewal and hope.*

Consequently, the latter part of *Av* is a time of rebuilding—both spiritually and physically. Even as Israel mourns its past failures, it also looks toward a future when repentance produces restoration and the fulfillment of God's promises.

The tribe of Simeon. The month of *Av* is associated with the tribe of Simeon, one of Jacob's twelve sons. Simeon was a mixed character, given to impulsive violence. For example, after their sister Dinah was violated, Simeon and his brother Levi exacted vengeance by slaughtering the men of Shechem (Genesis 34). This act of uncontrolled retribution resulted in Jacob cursing Simeon (Genesis 49:5-7).

This theme of uncontrolled emotion and the consequences that follow, form a spiritual thread of connection between the month of *Av* and the tribe of Simeon. In fact, Simeon's rash behavior mirrors the national sins of Israel that ultimately led to the Temple's destruction. Marty Solomon also draws parallels between Simeon's actions and how Israel's unfaithfulness and lack of discipline led to catastrophic events like those commemorated in *Av*.

Despite the fact that the tribe of Simeon does not play a prominent role in the future of Israel, the larger theme of *Av* demonstrates that the *hope for transformation and renewal is still possible*...even from the ashes of destruction. God called the nation of Israel (as well as Simeon), to confront its past, repent, and seek reconciliation with Him.

The letter Tet. *Av* is associated with the Hebrew letter *Tet* ["good"] whose numerical value of nine symbolizes judgment or fruitfulness. Traditionally, *Tet* is a paradoxical letter as it can represent either good or evil, depending on the context. The letter's physical shape suggests something concealed or curled inward, indicating that hidden potential lies within adversity.

The letter *Tet's* association with *Av* suggests the month's dual nature, holding potential for both destruction and rebirth. The hidden providence symbolized by *Tet* reminds us that God's goodness can emerge even in the darkest times.

This theme is confirmed by Dr. Michael S. Heiser, who notes that judgment often leads to restoration, with hidden blessings emerging from moments of crisis. Although the 9th of *Av* (*Tisha B'Av*) represents an historic day of catastrophic judgment, it also marks the beginning of the transition toward comfort and consolation.

The number five. *Av*, as the fifth month of the Hebrew calendar, is associated with the number five (5) which represents God's grace, provision, and responsibility. During *Av*, the number five assumes deeper layers of meaning, particularly in relation to the events of national judgment and restoration.

According to Dr. Michael S. Heiser, biblical numbers signify judgment and grace; in *Av*—a month of sorrow—people are called to both reflect on their sins and to seek God's mercy.

For Marty Solomon, the number five represents human responsibility in responding to God's grace, as seen in the aftermath of the temple's destruction, when Israel was called to *repent and rebuild*.

The number five also serves to remind us of (1) Israel's covenantal responsibility to maintain their relationship with God and (2) God's infinite grace in offering future restoration.

In addition to the number five, the number nine also plays a significant role in the month of *Av* due to its association with *Tisha B'Av* [9th day of *Av*]. In Scripture, nine usually represents finality or judgment.

For example, the ninth plague was darkness, a precursor to the final judgment which resulted in the death of Egypt's firstborn sons (Exodus 10:21-29).

This culmination of judgment is also illustrated by the fact that both Temples were destroyed on the same calendar day to demonstrate the finality of God's punishment for covenantal unfaithfulness. Yet, as previously noted, the number nine also carries the potential for new beginnings which is why, following *Tisha B'Av*, the focus shifts toward consolation and the hope of renewal.

According to Dr. G. K. Beale, the 9th day of *Av* marks the close of one chapter and the beginning of another, where repentance opens the door to divine mercy and healing.

The constellation Leo. *Av* is associated with the constellation of Leo [Heb. *Aryeh*] which is symbolized by the lion who represents strength, majesty, and sometimes destruction. The tribe of Judah is linked to the lion (Genesis 49:9) whose image can represent God's sovereignty and His judgment.

In the spiritual context of *Av*, Leo embodies both the fierceness of God's judgment and His eventual triumph. For example, the destruction of the Temple is a manifestation of God's righteous anger, but the lion also represents the Messianic hope of a future king from the line of David (the "Lion of Judah") who will restore Israel.

According to Marty Solomon, the lion illustrates the tension between God's judgment and mercy as it demonstrates how His fierce judgment is tempered by His covenantal promises of restoration.

Leo's connection to *Av* reminds us that while God's judgment can be painful, *His ultimate goal is to bring about justice and renewal*. Although the lion is a fearsome creature, it symbolizes the strength that God uses to restore His people in the Messianic age.

Spiritual focus during Av. The month of *Av* is a time of reflection, mourning, and hope. It reminds us that while there are consequences to covenantal unfaithfulness, God also offers us the renewal and restoration that follows repentance.

Followers of Yeshua are called to earnestly seek the renewal and comfort that comes through God's mercy and faithfulness.

Alignment in Av. The reason we process each month is to remain in alignment with God's rhythm of life. This means that we fearlessly examine both the good and the bad that happened each month to know where to invite God for healing, encouragement, direction, blessing, or repentance.

We believe that *unresolved grief is undelivered communication of an emotional nature.* When these communications (either positive or negative) are identified and expressed...*we experience emotional completion*. This enables us to keep our our hearts *clear* and *connected* as we practice alignment with God...instead of carrying our wounds and burdens into the next month.

Here's how we're going to use the Graphing Tool on the following pages:

STEP NO. 1: On the graph, start at the **BEGINNING OF MONTH** and continue to the **END OF MONTH**...

- Write down any events that happened, with positive events above the line and negative events below the line.
- Draw a line to represent the intensity of the event (the longer the line, the greater the intensity).
- Label each event with one of these emotional components:
  A = Apology • F = Forgive • S = Significant Emotional Statement

STEP NO. 2: Write out a **Significant Emotional Statement** for each event. This represents your emotional truth about how this event affected you. Some events can also have an **Apology** or a **Forgive** included in the statement and might be addressed to God, to another person, or even to yourself.

Reflect on the past month and write out (1) anything you need to apologize for, (2) anything you need to forgive, and (3) anything that describes your emotional truth. (Remember there is no judgment here...this is just for your heart to be clear, so be honest!)

STEP NO. 3: Write down anything that comes to your mind when you reflect on how God has shown up in these events.

In our monthly *Zoom Coaching* call, Inspired Life members will read their sentences and connections to their partner.

THE HEBREW MONTHS

END OF MONTH

STEP NO. 1

A = Apologies • F = Forgives • SES = Positive Significant Emotional Statements

Positive is above the line | **Negative** is below the line

BEGINNING OF MONTH

STEP NO. 2

A = Apologies

F = Forgives

SES = Positive Significant Emotional Statements

STEP NO. 3

REFLECTION: How did you see God move in the events of this month? (If this is hard to see, ask Him to help you interpret the events).

06 Elul | August – September

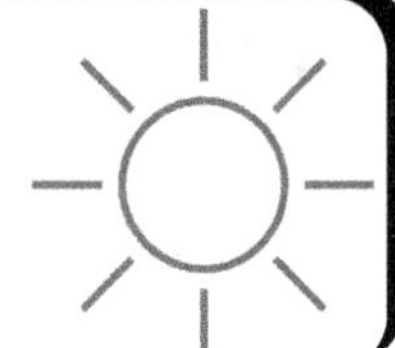

TRIBE	ALPHABET	NUMBER	CONSTELLATION
Gad	*YOD*	6	Virgo

Jacob + Zilpah = Gad

GENESIS 30:9-11 CJB | [9] When Le'ah saw that she had stopped having children, she took Zilpah her slave-girl and gave her to Ya'akov [Jacob] as his wife. [10] Zilpah, Le'ah's slave-girl bore Ya'akov a son; [11] and Le'ah said, "Good fortune has come," calling him Gad [good fortune].

The Blessing Of Jacob...

GENESIS 49:19 CJB | [19] "Gad [troop]— a troop will troop on him, but he will troop on their heel.

The Blessing Of Moses...

DEUTERONOMY 33:20-21 CJB | [20] Of Gad he said: "Blessed is he who makes Gad so large; he lies there like a lion, tearing arm and scalp. [21] He chose the best for himself when the princely portion was assigned. When the leaders of the people came, he carried out ADONAI's justice and his rulings concerning Isra'el."

NOTE: Due to the brevity of Jacob's blessing, it is admittedly difficult to link to any direct fulfillment in Scripture, although some Old Testament scholars believe this prophetic declaration was satisfied by the large number of troops from the tribe of Gad who served King David. (1 Chronicles 12).

Historical and biblical context. The Hebrew month of *Elul* is traditionally a time of self-examination, repentance, and spiritual preparation leading up to the High Holy Days of *Rosh Hashanah* and *Yom Kippur*.

Elul is known as the month of *teshuvah* ["repentance"] when individuals are called to consider their actions and seek reconciliation with God and others. In Jewish tradition, the *shofar* ["ram's horn"] is blown each day of the month to wake up the soul and encourage believers to return to God.

According to Marty Solomon, the seasonal rhythms of repentance recorded in Scripture reinforce the ways in which *Elul* provides a "spiritual reset" after the challenges and failures of the previous year.

This time of repentance is also connected to the story of Moses climbing Mount Sinai for the second time to receive the second set of tablets after Israel worshipped the Golden Calf during his first absence (Exodus 34:1-4).

According to Jewish tradition, Moses ascended on the first day of *Elul* and returned on *Yom Kippur*, forty days later. This underscores the month of *Elul* as a time of second chances and divine forgiveness.

Elul is also a time of spiritual preparation for the intense purification process of the "Ten Days of Awe" that take place between *Rosh Hashanah* and *Yom Kippur*. The cleansing of the soul during *Elul* prepares individuals for the new beginning ushered in by *Rosh Hashanah*, the Jewish New Year.

According to Dr. Michael S. Heiser, the biblical blueprint of repentance always precedes renewal, and *Elul* comports well with this pattern as it leads into the covenantal renewal celebrated during the High Holy Days.

A well-known rabbinic phrase describing *Elul* is *Ani L'dodi V'dodi Li* ["I am my beloved's, and my beloved is mine"] from the Song of Solomon (6:3). This phrase is often recited to express the intimate relationship between God and Israel during this time of year when God is seen as especially accessible to His people.

According to Marty Solomon, the covenantal relationship between God and Israel emphasizes *Elul* as a time when His presence feels nearer, and He invites us into personal transformation and intimacy.

The tribe of Gad. The month of *Elul* is associated with the tribe of Gad, one of Jacob's twelve sons. Gad's name means "good fortune" or "troop" (Genesis 30:11) and reflects his identity as a warrior tribe known for its military prowess (1 Chronicles 12:8).

The tribe of Gad symbolizes strength, preparation, and readiness for battle. In the context of *Elul*, this can be metaphorically understood as spiritual preparation for the coming High Holy Days.

Just as the tribe of Gad was well-prepared for physical battle, *Elul* calls us to prepare for spiritual battles of repentance, reflection, and reconciliation. This month inspires us to examine our actions and attitudes, strengthen our relationship with God, and ready ourselves for the spiritual renewal of *Rosh Hashanah* and *Yom Kippur*.

The letter Yod. *Elul* is associated with the Hebrew letter *Yod*, the smallest letter in the Hebrew alphabet. Despite its diminutive size, *Yod* represents "divine presence" and "humility". It is the first letter of *Yahweh's* name and represents His intimate and active involvement in the world. In *Elul*, the letter *Yod* reflects the humble posture that we are encouraged to adopt as we seek repentance and draw closer to God.

According to Dr. Michael S. Heiser, God's presence manifests in both the "macro" and the "micro" as the letter *Yod* reflects this theme of "divine nearness" during *Elul*. Consequently, we are encouraged to humble ourselves before God, acknowledge our shortcomings, and trust ourselves to His immeasurable mercy and grace.

The number six. *Elul*, as the sixth month of the Hebrew calendar, is associated with the number six (6) which represents "completion" or "work". For example, six days of creation (work) culminated in the seventh day of rest (Genesis 1-2). Therefore, six represents the final phase before completion, with a focus on preparation for the Sabbath rest.

This is why *Elul* is seen as a month of "spiritual work" in preparation for the rest and renewal offered during the High Holy Days. It is a time to assess one's actions, reconcile with others, and prepare for the culmination of the year.

According to Dr. G. K. Beale, biblical numbers can symbolize the spiritual process that calls believers to put in the "work of repentance" before entering the promised rest of God's covenantal renewal. In other words, since God can't repent for us...we must seek the restoration and healing of our union with Him.

The constellation Virgo. *Elul* is associated with the constellation of Virgo [Heb. *Betulah*] which means "virgin". In Jewish tradition, the virgin represents purity, innocence, and new beginnings. *Elul*, as a month of repentance, reflects these qualities by calling for spiritual purification in preparation for the renewal of the new year.

According to Marty Solomon, spiritual renewal and the opportunity for new beginnings is one of the central themes of *Elul*. He further noted that the constellation of Virgo, symbolizing virginal purity, aligns with the month's focus on spiritual cleansing and the "opportunity to start fresh."

Additionally, Virgo can be understood to represent Israel as God's beloved bride in prophetic literature, where His relationship with His people is often compared to a marital bond (e.g., Hosea, Jeremiah, et. al.). Thus, *Elul* is a time of relational renewal as we return to God with a pure heart.

Spiritual focus during Elul. The month of *Elul* is a time for reflection, repentance, and preparation. It also embodies a season of self-examination when we confront our sins and seek reconciliation with both God and others. This "spiritual work" is critical in preparing for the High Holy Days.

Alignment in Elul. The reason we process each month is to remain in alignment with God's rhythm of life. This means that we fearlessly examine both the good and the bad that happened each month to know where to invite God for healing, encouragement, direction, blessing, or repentance.

We believe that *unresolved grief is undelivered communication of an emotional nature.* When these communications (either positive or negative) are identified and expressed...*we experience emotional completion*. This enables us to keep our our hearts *clear* and *connected* as we practice alignment with God...instead of carrying our wounds and burdens into the next month.

Here's how we're going to use the Graphing Tool on the following pages:

STEP NO. 1: On the graph, start at the **BEGINNING OF MONTH** and continue to the **END OF MONTH**...

- Write down any events that happened, with positive events above the line and negative events below the line.
- Draw a line to represent the intensity of the event (the longer the line, the greater the intensity).
- Label each event with one of these emotional components:
  A = Apology • F = Forgive • S = Significant Emotional Statement

STEP NO. 2: Write out a **Significant Emotional Statement** for each event. This represents your emotional truth about how this event affected you. Some events can also have an **Apology** or a **Forgive** included in the statement and might be addressed to God, to another person, or even to yourself.

Reflect on the past month and write out (1) anything you need to apologize for, (2) anything you need to forgive, and (3) anything that describes your emotional truth. (Remember there is no judgment here...this is just for your heart to be clear, so be honest!)

STEP NO. 3: Write down anything that comes to your mind when you reflect on how God has shown up in these events.

In our monthly *Zoom Coaching* call, Inspired Life members will read their sentences and connections to their partner.

THE HEBREW MONTHS

END OF MONTH

STEP NO. 1

A = Apologies • F = Forgives • SES = Positive Significant Emotional Statements

Positive is above the line | **Negative** is below the line

BEGINNING OF MONTH

STEP NO. 2

A = Apologies

F = Forgives

SES = Positive Significant Emotional Statements

REFLECTION: How did you see God move in the events of this month? (If this is hard to see, ask Him to help you interpret the events).

STEP NO. 3

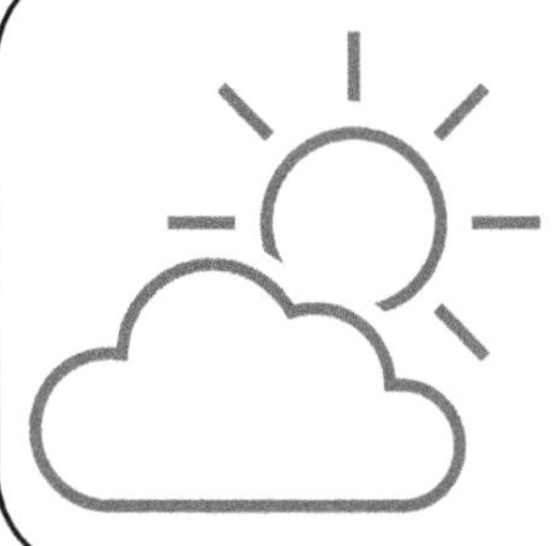

AUTUMN | **Tishrei**

7 Tishrei | September – October
8 Cheshvan | October – November
9 Kislev | November – December

Autumn [Heb. Stav] is a season of harvest completion, celebration, and reflection. Agriculturally, it is when the final ingathering of crops occurs, especially the fruit harvest, which is marked by the festival of Sukkot [Feast of Tabernacles]. This festival celebrates both God's provision during the Israelites' wilderness journey and the blessings of the completed harvest.

Spiritually, autumn is a season of repentance and renewal. It begins with the High Holy Days of Rosh Hashanah [Jewish New Year] and Yom Kippur [Day of Atonement], when individuals reflect on their lives, seek atonement, and renew their relationship with God.

According to Marty Solomon, autumn is a time of evaluation, when believers assess the spiritual fruit of the past year and commit to spiritual renewal. Dr. G. K. Beale has further noted that these festivals prefigure themes of eschatological judgment and restoration, with Sukkot pointing toward the ultimate ingathering of God's people in the Messianic age.

Thus, autumn is a season of joyful thanksgiving, spiritual reflection, and preparation for the new cycle of growth.

7 Tishrei ["early rains, plowing"] • **8 Cheshvan** ["wheat, barley sowing"] • **9 Kislev** [Nehemiah 1:1; Zechariah 7:1]

NOTE: Some scholars associate *Kislev* with the word *ksil* ["fool"] demonstrating the depth of God's love…even for those who have acted foolishly. (Ezra 10)

07 Tishrei | September – October

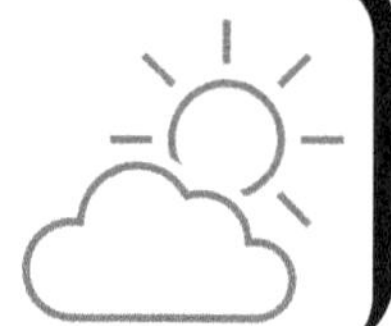

TRIBE	ALPHABET	NUMBER	CONSTELLAATION
Ephraim	*LAMED*	7	Libra

Jacob + Rachel = Joseph ↪Joseph + Asenath = Ephraim

GENESIS 30:22-24 CJB | 22 Then God took note of Rachel, heeded her prayer and made her fertile. 23 She conceived, had a son and said, "God has taken away my disgrace." 24 She called him Yosef [may he add], saying, "May ADONAI add to me another son."

The Blessing Of Jacob…

GENESIS 49:22-26 CJB | 22 "Yosef [Joseph] is a fruitful plant, a fruitful plant by a spring, with branches climbing over the wall. 23 The archers attacked him fiercely, shooting at him and pressing him hard; 24 but his bow remained taut; and his arms were made nimble by the hands of the Mighty One of Ya'akov [Jacob], from there, from the Shepherd, the Stone of Isra'el, 25 by the God of your father, who will help you, by El Shaddai [Almighty], who will bless you with blessings from heaven above, blessings from the deep, lying below, blessings from the breasts and the womb. 26 The blessings of your father are more powerful than the blessings of my parents, extending to the farthest of the everlasting hills; they will be on the head of Yosef, on the brow of the prince among his brothers.

The Blessing Of Moses…

DEUTERONOMY 33:13-17 CJB | 13 Of Yosef he said: "May ADONAI bless his

land with the best from the sky, for the dew, and for what comes from the
deep beneath, [14] with the best of what the sun makes grow, with the best of
what comes up each month, [15] with the best from the mountains of old, with
the best from the eternal hills, [16] with the best from the earth and all that fills it,
and the favor of him who lived in the [burning] bush. May blessing come on
the head of Yosef, on the brow of the prince among his brothers. [17] His
firstborn bull — glory is his; his horns are those of a wild ox; With them he will
gore the peoples, all of them, to the ends of the earth. These are the myriads
of Efrayim [Ephraim]; these are the thousands of M'nasheh [Manasseh]."

Historical and biblical context. The Hebrew month of *Tishrei* marks the beginning of the new year and is packed with pivotal events and festivals such as *Rosh Hashanah*, *Yom Kippur*, and *Sukkot*.

Tishrei is best known for its connection to *Rosh Hashanah* [Jewish New Year], when, according to Hebrew tradition, God judges all of creation. It starts with the "Days of Awe", a ten-day period of repentance, and culminates in *Yom Kippur* ["Day of Atonement"], the holiest day of the year.

According to Marty Solomon, this month is connected to themes of reflection and reconciliation…both with God and within the Messianic community.

According to Dr. Michael S. Heiser, *Tishrei* is the month when God's covenant with Israel was reaffirmed, and the people were then called to account for their actions from the previous year. *Rosh Hashanah* and *Yom Kippur* both point to God's sovereignty over creation and His relentless desire to restore the relationship between Himself and His people.

Following *Yom Kippur*, the festival of *Sukkot* ["Feast of Tabernacles"] celebrates God's provision and remembers Israel's time in the wilderness, when He dwelled among His people in the Tabernacle. *Sukkot* honors God's enduring faithfulness and invites us to rejoice in His presence.

According to Dr. G. K. Beale, since this festival commemorates when God dwelt among His people in the wilderness, it points to the future when He will dwell with His people in the final restoration of the world.

Sukkot is also a time of thanksgiving for the fall harvest as it reminds us of God's continual provision. The temporary *sukkah* ["booth"] built during this time also recalls the transient nature of human life and our total dependence on God's care. This festival, like the other *Tishrei* celebrations, emphasizes the covenantal relationship between God and Israel.

In addition to its spiritual importance, *Tishrei* marks the beginning of the agricultural year in ancient Israel. This was the time of the final fruit harvest, especially grapes and olives, as the land was prepared for a new agricultural cycle.

According to Marty Solomon, the agricultural rhythms described in Scripture also reflect cycles of spiritual completion and renewal. During *Tishrei*, these rhythms link the physical and spiritual realms to give us a powerful model of *growth and rebirth...completion and renewal*.

The tribe of Ephraim. The month of *Tishrei* is associated with the tribe of Ephraim, one of Joseph's two sons. Ephraim means "fruitfulness" (Genesis 41:52) and his name aligns with the harvest season of *Tishrei*, a time of ingathering and abundance, both agriculturally and spiritually.

Ephraim was one of the prominent tribes in Israel's northern kingdom, often representing the strength and potential of God's people. In the context of *Tishrei*, this illustrates the importance of spiritual fruitfulness (i.e., our need to produce the fruits of repentance, righteousness, and obedience to God's covenant).

The tribe of Ephraim also faced warnings and judgments from the prophets (Hosea 4:17) for its disobedience which mirrors the themes of repentance and renewal that *Tishrei* embodies.

The letter Lamed. *Tishrei* is associated with the Hebrew letter *Lamed*, which is also the tallest letter in the Hebrew alphabet. *Lamed* represents learning, teaching, and leadership, highlighting Israel's role as a light to the nations during this season of spiritual reflection and repentance.

The shape of *Lamed* resembles a staff or goad, symbolizing guidance and direction. Both of these themes feature prominently in the festivals held during *Tishrei*, when the people are reminded of God's judgment, mercy, and ultimate redemption. Each festival emphasizes God's call on the Messianic community to seek His wisdom and align with His will.

According to Marty Solomon, the letter *Lamed*, symbolizing learning, connects to *Tishrei's* reflective nature—a month that invites us to learn from past mistakes and recommit to God's teachings for the year ahead.

The number seven. *Tishrei*, as the seventh month of the Hebrew calendar, is associated with the number seven (7) and represents completion, perfection, and rest. Just as God created the world in six days and rested on the seventh (Genesis 2:2-3), *Tishrei* is a time of spiritual completion and renewal.

The three festivals in *Tishrei* (*Rosh Hashanah*, *Yom Kippur*, and *Sukkot*) are all connected to the themes of completion, judgment, and rest. *Yom Kippur*, in particular, reflects the completion of the atonement process when God's people are cleansed and made right with Him.

According to Dr. Michael J. Heiser, the number seven signifies divine order and the restoration of relationships, particularly in the context of covenant relationships.

The seventh month mirrors the Sabbath rest promised in God's kingdom, a time of ultimate completion when we'll be fully restored to live in harmony with Him.

The constellation Libra. *Tishrei* is associated with the constellation of Libra [Heb. *Moznayim*] which means "scales." In Jewish tradition, the scales represent judgment, and this symbol perfectly aligns with the judgment themes of *Tishrei* (e.g., *Rosh Hashanah* and *Yom Kippur* are understood as times when God "weighs" the actions of humanity and determines their destiny for the coming year.

The scales of Libra remind us of the balance between justice and mercy...

judgment and forgiveness. As we reflect on our actions and seek repentance during this month, we remember the delicate balance between God's righteousness and His grace. Thus, the scales symbolize both accountability and the potential for redemption.

Spiritual focus during Tishrei. Through repentance and reconciliation…with God, ourselves, and others…we are called to seek "fruitfulness" that leads to renewal in our relationship with Him and with the people in our lives.

As we remember God's provision, both past and present, we assume a posture of gratitude as we look forward to a fresh start for the coming year.

> **ISAIAH 43:19 CJB** | [19] I am doing something new; it's springing up — can't you see it? I am making a road in the desert, rivers in the wasteland.

> **REVELATION 21:5 CJB** | [5] Then the One sitting on the throne said, "Look! I am making everything new!" Also, he said, "Write, 'These words are true and trustworthy!'"

Ultimately, God wants us to experience His presence, and these festivals offer an incredible opportunity to intentionally set aside time to assess what He is teaching us and how we can deepen our union with Him.

Alignment in Tishrei. The reason we process each month is to remain in alignment with God's rhythm of life. This means that we fearlessly examine both the good and the bad that happened each month to know where to invite God for healing, encouragement, direction, blessing, or repentance.

We believe that *unresolved grief is undelivered communication of an emotional nature.* When these communications (either positive or negative) are identified and expressed...*we experience emotional completion*. This enables us to keep our our hearts *clear* and *connected* as we practice alignment with God...instead of carrying our wounds and burdens into the next month.

Here's how we're going to use the Graphing Tool on the following pages:

STEP NO. 1: On the graph, start at the **BEGINNING OF MONTH** and continue to the **END OF MONTH**...

- Write down any events that happened, with positive events above the line and negative events below the line.
- Draw a line to represent the intensity of the event (the longer the line, the greater the intensity).
- Label each event with one of these emotional components:
  A = Apology • F = Forgive • S = Significant Emotional Statement

STEP NO. 2: Write out a **Significant Emotional Statement** for each event. This represents your emotional truth about how this event affected you. Some events can also have an **Apology** or a **Forgive** included in the statement and might be addressed to God, to another person, or even to yourself.

Reflect on the past month and write out (1) anything you need to apologize for, (2) anything you need to forgive, and (3) anything that describes your emotional truth. (Remember there is no judgment here...this is just for your heart to be clear, so be honest!)

STEP NO. 3: Write down anything that comes to your mind when you reflect on how God has shown up in these events.

In our monthly *Zoom Coaching* call, Inspired Life members will read their sentences and connections to their partner.

THE HEBREW MONTHS

END OF MONTH

STEP NO. 1

A = Apologies • F = Forgives • SES = Positive Significant Emotional Statements

Positive is above the line | **Negative** is below the line

BEGINNING OF MONTH

STEP NO. 2

A = Apologies

F = Forgives

SES = Positive Significant Emotional Statements

REFLECTION: How did you see God move in the events of this month? (If this is hard to see, ask Him to help you interpret the events).

STEP NO. 3

08 Cheshvan | October – November

TRIBE	ALPHABET	NUMBER	CONSTELLATION
Manasseh	*NUN*	8	Scorpio

Jacob + Rachel = Joseph ↪Joseph + Asenath = Manasseh

The Blessing Of Jacob…

GENESIS 48:1-6 CJB | 1 Awhile later someone told Yosef [Joseph] that his father
was ill. He took with him his two sons, M'nasheh [Manasseh] and Efrayim
[Ephraim]. 2 Ya'akov [Jacob] was told, "Here comes your son Yosef."

Isra'el [Jacob] gathered his strength and sat up in bed. 3 Ya'akov [Jacob] said
to Yosef [Joseph], "El Shaddai [Almighty] appeared to me at Luz in the land of
Kena'an [Canaan] and blessed me, 4 saying to me, 'I will make you fruitful and
numerous. I will make of you a group of peoples; and I will give this land to
your descendants to possess forever.' 5 Now your two sons, who were born
to you in the land of Egypt before I came to you in Egypt, are mine; Efrayim
[Ephraim] and M'nasheh [Manasseh] will be as much mine as Re'uven
[Reuben] and Shim'on [Simeon] are. 6 The children born to you after them will
be yours, but for purposes of inheritance they are to be counted with their
older brothers.

The Blessing Of Moses…

DEUTERONOMY 33:16-17 CJB | 16 […] May blessing come on the head of Yosef
[Joseph], on the brow of the prince among his brothers. 17 His firstborn bull —
glory is his; his horns are those of a wild ox; with them he will gore the peoples

all of them, to the ends of the earth. These are the myriads of Efrayim [Ephraim]; these are the thousands of M'nasheh [Manasseh]."

Historical and biblical context. The Hebrew month of *Cheshvan* is uniquely notable for the absence of festivals and stands out in sharp contrast to the spiritually charged month of *Tishrei*. which features *Rosh Hashanah, Yom Kippur*, and the week-long festival of *Sukkot*. Due to this lack of celebration, it is sometimes referred to as *Mar-Cheshvan* ["bitter month"], though it remains historically and spiritually significant.

In Hebrew tradition, this is a time of quiet reflection and continued focus on everyday faithfulness, as one returns to the normal rhythms of life following the high holidays of *Tishrei*.

According to Marty Solomon, the absence of festivals in *Cheshvan* allows for an opportunity to internalize the lessons learned during *Tishrei*, especially in the areas of repentance and renewal.

Thus, *Cheshvan* invites us to return to normal life and to live out the values of repentance, faithfulness, and devotion in our day-to-day actions. According to Dr. Michael S. Heiser, these periods of calm allow us to focus on cultivating a lasting union with God, not just during special celebrations.

In ancient Israel, *Cheshvan* was a key month in the agricultural cycle because it marked the the beginning of the rainy season. Following the harvest festivals of *Tishrei*, the people of Israel customarily began praying for the life-giving rains that ensured the success of the next year's crops. These prayers were for God's provision and faithfulness and today they remind us that even during times of stillness and inactivity, God's care is constant...and necessary.

This agricultural focus highlights the deeper importance of waiting on God. As the rain comes, it symbolizes His nourishment and the promise that He will sustain us even during times that seem spiritually barren.

According to Hebrew scholars, the Great Flood in the days of Noah began during the month of *Cheshvan*. Though a somber historical element representing God's judgment, it also reminds us of His covenant with Noah afterward, symbolized by the rainbow. In a larger sense, the flood narrative illustrates God's sovereignty over creation, His willingness to bring judgment, but also His merciful promise to preserve humanity.

According to Dr. G. K. Beale's study of covenants in Scripture, God's covenant with Noah after the flood represented His continued faithfulness to humanity, even during times of judgment. This connection further demonstrates the themes of reflection and trust in God's mercy that is encouraged during *Cheshvan*.

The tribe of Manasseh. The month of *Cheshvan* is associated with the tribe of Manasseh, one of Joseph's two sons. Manasseh's name means "to forget" (Genesis 41:51), as Joseph named him to honor how God helped him forget his troubles and hardships in Egypt.

The connection to Manasseh reflects the quiet nature of *Cheshvan*—a month that follows intense spiritual work of *Tishrei*—when past burdens are released. Just as Manasseh was a tribe marked by growth and healing; *Cheshvan* likewise invites us to release our past struggles as we look toward the future with renewed hope.

The letter Nun. *Cheshvan* is associated with the letter *Nun* which represents humility and faithfulness. In its final form, *Nun* extends downward, symbolizing someone who is bent low in humility before God.

This relationship with humility seamlessly blends into the quiet and reflective nature of *Cheshvan*, as we are called to continue in faithfulness and humility without the external celebrations or rituals of the prior months. As Marty Solomon has wisely observed, spiritual growth often happens in the ordinary, quiet moments of life.

The letter *Nun* can also symbolize continuity, reflecting that even in times of spiritual quietness, God's covenantal promises and care remain constant and unbroken.

The number eight. *Cheshvan*, as the eighth month of the Hebrew calendar, is associated with the number eight (8) which represents new beginnings and renewal. The number eight extends past the completeness of seven to transcend the natural order. For example, circumcision is performed on the eighth day (Genesis 17:12) as a sign of the covenant between God and Israel and symbolizes a new beginning in the life of the child.

The number eight's association with new beginnings reflects this promise of growth and renewal during the month of *Cheshvan*. It is a time when God is quietly preparing something new, much like the rains that fall during *Cheshvan* prepare the land for new life in the spring season.

According to Dr. Michael S. Heiser, the number eight signifies hope and restoration and is closely related to how the month of *Cheshvan* appears quiet even as it holds the promise of future growth.

The constellation Scorpio. *Cheshvan* is associated with the constellation of Scorpio [Heb. *Akrav*] which means "scorpion." In Jewish tradition, scorpions symbolize testing and challenge (Deuteronomy 8:15) and remind us of the dangers and hardships that we face in life.

Scorpio's connection to *Cheshvan* also reflects the hidden challenges of the month, as the people of Israel transitioned from the spiritual highs of *Tishrei* to the more subdued, less celebrated period of *Cheshvan*. The scorpion's sting serves as a metaphor for spiritual vigilance, reminding us to remain faithful and humble even when there are no external reminders or festivals to keep us focused.

According to Marty Solomon, periods of both serenity and testing are crucial for spiritual growth, as they encourage us to place our trust in God rather than rituals or community reinforcement.

Spiritual focus during Cheshvan. Absent the high-profile holidays of other months, *Cheshvan* is a time to daily live out our trust in God. It is a time to partner with Him in quiet humility and remain vigilant as we prepare for a season of spiritual growth in the face of unknown challenges.

Alignment in Cheshvan. The reason we process each month is to remain in alignment with God's rhythm of life. This means that we fearlessly examine both the good and the bad that happened each month to know where to invite God for healing, encouragement, direction, blessing, or repentance.

We believe that *unresolved grief is undelivered communication of an emotional nature.* When these communications (either positive or negative) are identified and expressed...*we experience emotional completion*. This enables us to keep our our hearts *clear* and *connected* as we practice alignment with God...instead of carrying our wounds and burdens into the next month.

Here's how we're going to use the Graphing Tool on the following pages:

STEP NO. 1: On the graph, start at the **BEGINNING OF MONTH** and continue to the **END OF MONTH**...

- Write down any events that happened, with positive events above the line and negative events below the line.
- Draw a line to represent the intensity of the event (the longer the line, the greater the intensity).
- Label each event with one of these emotional components:
  A = Apology • F = Forgive • S = Significant Emotional Statement

STEP NO. 2: Write out a **Significant Emotional Statement** for each event. This represents your emotional truth about how this event affected you. Some events can also have an **Apology** or a **Forgive** included in the statement and might be addressed to God, to another person, or even to yourself.

Reflect on the past month and write out (1) anything you need to apologize for, (2) anything you need to forgive, and (3) anything that describes your emotional truth. (Remember there is no judgment here...this is just for your heart to be clear, so be honest!)

STEP NO. 3: Write down anything that comes to your mind when you reflect on how God has shown up in these events.

In our monthly *Zoom Coaching* call, Inspired Life members will read their sentences and connections to their partner.

THE HEBREW MONTHS

END OF MONTH

STEP NO. 1

A = Apologies • F = Forgives • SES = Positive Significant Emotional Statements
Positive is above the line | **Negative** is below the line

BEGINNING OF MONTH

STEP NO. 2

A = Apologies

F = Forgives

SES = Positive Significant Emotional Statements

REFLECTION: How did you see God move in the events of this month? (If this is hard to see, ask Him to help you interpret the events).

STEP NO. 3

09 Kislev | November – December

TRIBE	ALPHABET	NUMBER	CONSTELLATION
Benjamin	*SAMEKH*	9	Sagittarius

Jacob + Rachel = Benjamin

GENESIS 35:17-18 CJB | 17 While she [Rachel] was undergoing this hard labor, the midwife said to her, "Don't worry, this is also a son for you." 18 But she died in childbirth. As she was dying, she named her son Ben-Oni [son of my grief], but his father called him Binyamin [son of the right hand, son of the south].

The Blessing Of Jacob…

GENESIS 49:27 CJB | 27 "Binyamin [Benjamin] is a ravenous wolf, in the morning devouring the prey, in the evening still dividing the spoil."

The Blessing Of Moses…

DEUTERONOMY 33:12 CJB | 12 Of Binyamin [Benjamin] he said: "ADONAI's beloved lives securely. He protects him day after day. He lives between his shoulders."

Historical and biblical context. The Hebrew month of *Kislev* is notable for being a time of light and hope, particularly since it is when the festival of *Hanukkah* is celebrated. *Kislev* is traditionally associated with themes of trust, security, and spiritual awakening amidst the darkness of the winter season.

Hanukkah is observed on the 25th of *Kislev* to commemorate the Maccabean Revolt (168-164 BC) and the miraculous re-dedication of the Temple in Jerusalem during the Second Temple period (516 BC-70 AD). The festival celebrates God's provision and protection of His people during a time of oppression and tyranny.

According to Marty Solomon, *Hanukkah* is a time of spiritual renewal and perseverance when the light of God's presence shines in the midst of political and spiritual challenges. The festival is marked by the lighting of the *menorah* which symbolizes the victory of light over physical and spiritual darkness.

In ancient Israel, *Kislev* was part of the early rainy season when the land receives the water necessary for future growth. The arrival of these rains is crucial for the agricultural cycle, and the people of Israel eagerly sought God's provision during this season.

The rains of *Kislev* represent physical nourishment for the land as well as a spiritual outpouring of God's faithfulness. Their reliance upon God to bring rain symbolized trusting in His broader provision and security...which also ties into the central themes of faith and hope.

In the *Torah*, *Kislev* is associated with the patriarch Joseph, whose ability to interpret dreams played a significant role in Scripture. In Genesis 37, Joseph's dreams, which likely happened during the season of *Kislev*, foreshadowed his rise to prominence in Egypt and the eventual rescue of his family during the great famine.

Joseph's incredible story of betrayal, imprisonment, and ascension to second-in-command in Egypt through God's provision, reflects *Kislev's* spiritual message: even in times of terrible darkness or uncertainty, God's purposes are at work. Thus, the dreams and visions associated with *Kislev* underscore the theme of divine revelation and guidance in the midst of trials.

The tribe of Benjamin. The month of Kislev is associated with the tribe of Benjamin, one of Jacob's twelve sons. Benjamin's name means "son of the right hand" or "son of strength" which symbolizes the protection and security that comes from God's presence.

Though the smallest of the twelve tribes, Benjamin held a pivotal role in Israel's history due to its strength, resilience, and possession of Jerusalem. In connection with *Kislev*, this forms another link to the month's theme of finding spiritual security and hope in God, even during the most desperate circumstances. According to Dr. G. K. Beale, this theme is amplified throughout Scripture in the way that God's presence offers divine protection and refuge for His people.

The letter Samekh. *Kislev* is associated with the letter *Samekh* whose enclosed circular form represents support, protection, and trust. The word *samekh* means to lean upon or to uphold which symbolizes God's continuous sustenance and support of His people.

Samekh's connection to *Kislev* highlights the month's larger theme of relying on God's protection in times of darkness. Just as the written form of *Samekh* encloses and surrounds, God's presence surrounds His people, offering them security when they are vulnerable.

According to Marty Solomon, trust plays an essential role, particularly in times when God's presence or purpose might not be immediately apparent. The letter *Samekh* reflects the deep trust in God's guidance and care that characterizes *Kislev*.

The number nine. *Kislev*, as the ninth month of the Hebrew calendar, is associated with the number nine (9) and represents completeness or finality, especially regarding judgment or divine activity. Nine also relates to the fruit of the Spirit, as there are nine specific attributes listed in the New Testament.

> **GALATIANS 5:22 CJB** | 22 But the fruit of the Spirit is love, joy, peace, patience, kindness, goodness, faithfulness, 23 humility, self-control. Nothing in the *Torah* stands against such things.

The number nine's connection to divine completeness also reflects the spiritual journey of *Kislev*: a period of trusting that God's purposes, though sometimes unseen, are coming to fulfillment. In this way, *Hanukkah* celebrates divine deliverance in Israel's victory over the Seleucid Greek Empire (312 BC-64 BC) and the fulfillment of God's promise in the Temple's restoration.

The constellation Sagittarius. *Kislev* is associated with the constellation of Sagittarius [Heb. *Keshet*] which means "bow." In Jewish tradition, *keshet* refers to both the rainbow and the archer's bow, with the former symbolizing God's covenant after the flood in the days of Noah (Genesis 9:13-17).

The rainbow, as a symbol of God's promise, ties into the themes of faithfulness and hope that infuse *Kislev*. The bow of Sagittarius symbolizes readiness for action and spiritual warfare, aligning with *Hanukkah's* celebration of the Maccabees' victory.

The bow also symbolizes God as Protector, who fights for His people just as He did during the events of *Hanukkah*. The imagery of the bow draws our attention to the importance of vigilance and trust that is required during *Kislev*...a season of physical and spiritual preparation.

Spiritual focus during Kislev. Although applicable whenever we lack trust in God to provide for our needs, this special window of *Kislev* can be a life-changing opportunity to become curious...to seek His presence...to partner with Him to get to the root of the mistrust and experience healing. When we choose to lean on God, in good times and bad, our trust in Him is strengthened. Thus, this is a month to be especially vigilant and ready for action while trusting in God's timing and deliverance.

Alignment in Kislev. The reason we process each month is to remain in alignment with God's rhythm of life. This means that we fearlessly examine both the good and the bad that happened each month to know where to invite God for healing, encouragement, direction, blessing, or repentance.

We believe that *unresolved grief is undelivered communication of an emotional nature.* When these communications (either positive or negative) are identified and expressed...*we experience emotional completion*. This enables us to keep our our hearts *clear* and *connected* as we practice alignment with God...instead of carrying our wounds and burdens into the next month.

Here's how we're going to use the Graphing Tool on the following pages:

STEP NO. 1: On the graph, start at the **BEGINNING OF MONTH** and continue to the **END OF MONTH**...

- Write down any events that happened, with positive events above the line and negative events below the line.
- Draw a line to represent the intensity of the event (the longer the line, the greater the intensity).
- Label each event with one of these emotional components:
  A = Apology • F = Forgive • S = Significant Emotional Statement

STEP NO. 2: Write out a **Significant Emotional Statement** for each event. This represents your emotional truth about how this event affected you. Some events can also have an **Apology** or a **Forgive** included in the statement and might be addressed to God, to another person, or even to yourself.

Reflect on the past month and write out (1) anything you need to apologize for, (2) anything you need to forgive, and (3) anything that describes your emotional truth. (Remember there is no judgment here...this is just for your heart to be clear, so be honest!)

STEP NO. 3: Write down anything that comes to your mind when you reflect on how God has shown up in these events.

In our monthly *Zoom Coaching* call, Inspired Life members will read their sentences and connections to their partner.

THE HEBREW MONTHS

END OF MONTH

STEP NO. 1

A = Apologies • F = Forgives • SES = Positive Significant Emotional Statements

Positive is above the line | **Negative** is below the line

BEGINNING OF MONTH

STEP NO. 2

A = Apologies

F = Forgives

SES = Positive Significant Emotional Statements

REFLECTION: How did you see God move in the events of this month? (If this is hard to see, ask Him to help you interpret the events).

STEP NO. 3

You might be wondering why the tribe of Levi was not included in the twelve months. They were unique among the other tribes of Israel in that they received no allotment of land from God. Instead, they were assigned other responsibilities.

> **NUMBERS 3:5-9 CJB** | [5] ADONAI said to Moshe [Moses], [6] "Summon the tribe of Levi, and assign them to Aharon [Aaron] the cohen [priest], so that they can help him. [7] They are to carry out his duties and the duties of the whole community before the tent of meeting in performing the service of the tabernacle. [8] They are to be in charge of all the furnishings of the tent of meeting and to carry out all the duties of the people of Isra'el connected with the service of the tabernacle. [9] Assign the L'vi'im [Levites] to Aharon and his sons; their one responsibility in regard to the people of Isra'el is to serve him.

The reason for God's assignment is found in verse 11...

> **NUMBERS 3:11-13 CJB** | [11] ADONAI said to Moshe [Moses], [12] "I have taken the L'vi'im [Levites] from among the people of Isra'el in lieu of every firstborn male that is first from the womb among the people of Isra'el; the L'vi'im are to be mine. [13] All the firstborn males belong to me, because on the day that I killed all the firstborn males in the land of Egypt, I separated for myself all the firstborn males in Isra'el, both human and animal. They are mine; I am ADONAI."

Thus, the tribe of Levi became a sacrifice of gratitude for God's deliverance from the Egyptians. In exchange for the firstborn males and livestock, God took the Levites as a sacrifice for Him and dedicated the tribe to His service.

Consequently, the tribe of Levi were not allocated their own territorial lands when the Israelites entered the Promised Land but instead, lived in the 48 Levitical cities set aside for their tribe. This arrangement enabled them to perform their priestly services throughout all of Canaan.

Jacob + Leah = Levi

> **GENESIS 29:34 CJB** | [34] Once more she [Leah] conceived and had a son; and

she said, "Now this time my husband [Jacob] will be joined to me, because I have borne him three sons." Therefore, she named him Levi [joining].

The Blessing Of Jacob...

GENESIS 49:5-7 CJB | 5 "Shim'on [Simeon] and Levi are brothers, related by weapons of violence. 6 Let me not enter their council, let my honor not be connected with their people; for in their anger, they killed men, and at their whim they maimed cattle. 7 Cursed be their anger, for it has been fierce; their fury, for it has been cruel. I will divide them in Ya'akov [Jacob] and scatter them in Isra'el.

The Blessing Of Moses...

DEUTERONOMY 33:8-11 CJB | 8 Of Levi he said: "Let your tumim and urim [breastplate] be with your pious one, whom you tested at Massah, with whom you struggled at M'rivah Spring. 9 Of his father and mother he said, 'I don't know them'; he didn't acknowledge his brothers or children. For he observed your word, and he kept your covenant. 10 They will teach Ya'akov [Jacob] your rulings, Isra'el your Torah [Law]. They will set incense before you and whole burnt offerings on your altar. 11 ADONAI, bless his possessions, accept the work he does; but crush his enemy's hip and thigh; may those who hate him rise no more."

Jacob grouped Simeon and Levi together because they exacted revenge against the men of Shechem for raping their sister, Dinah (Genesis 34:27-29). What they did not plunder, they apparently destroyed and were therefore divided and scattered as punishment.

Levi also means "attached" or "joined," and was the tribe chosen to serve in the Temple. Thus, Levi represents the dedication of your life to serving a higher calling, freeing yourself from being bound to material survival, and attaching yourself to the service of God.

THE APPPOINTED TIMES

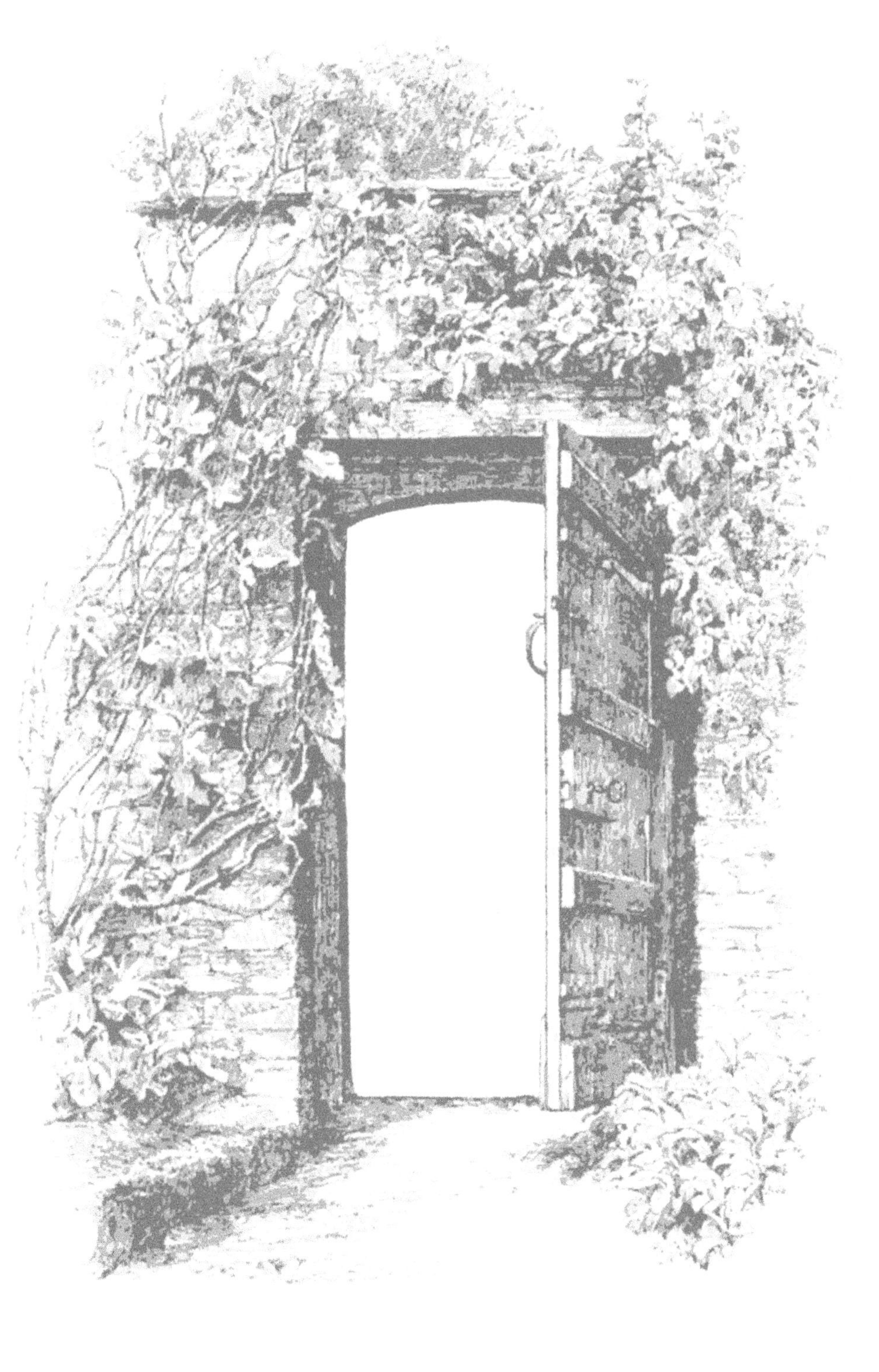

Part 5

THE APPPOINTED TIMES

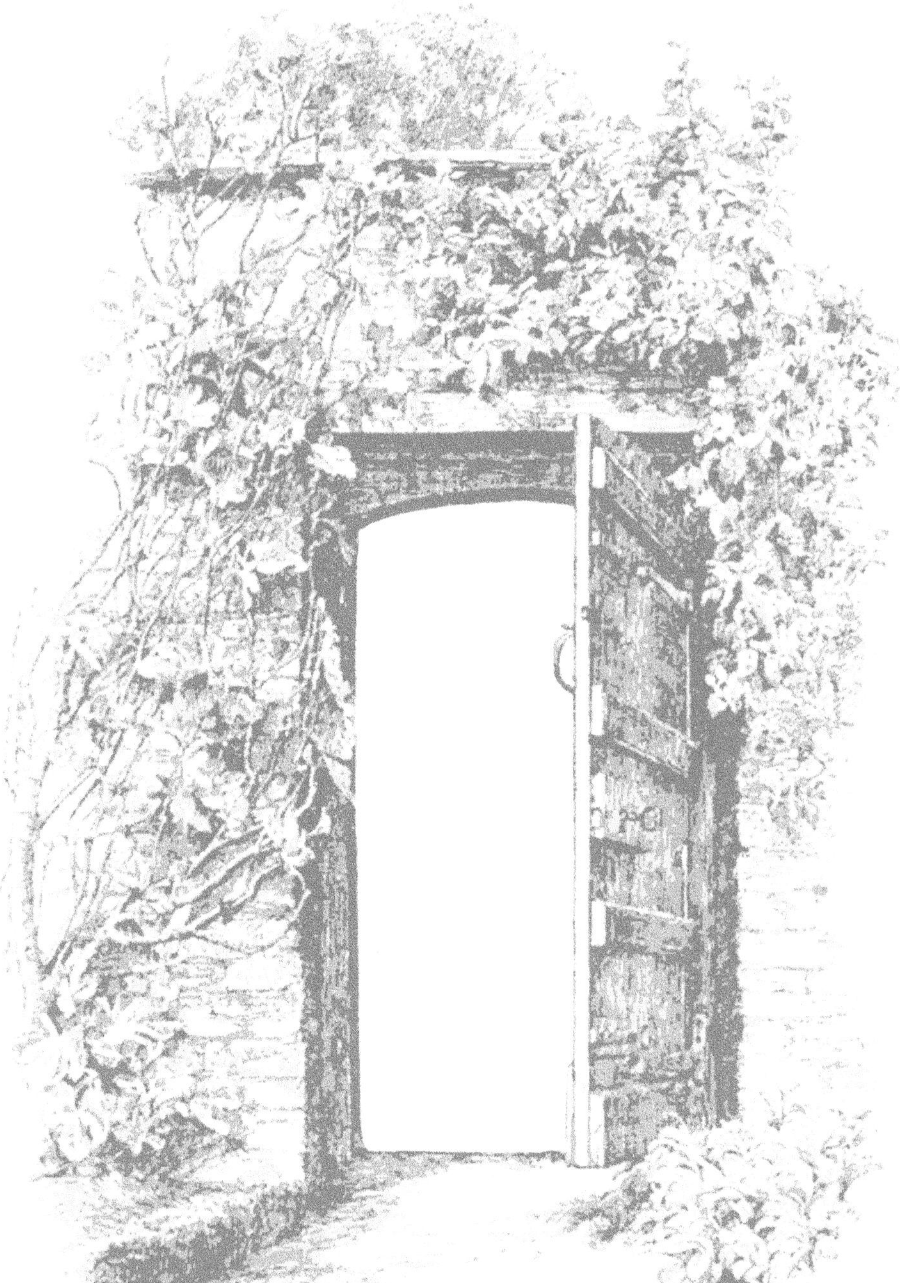

Part 5

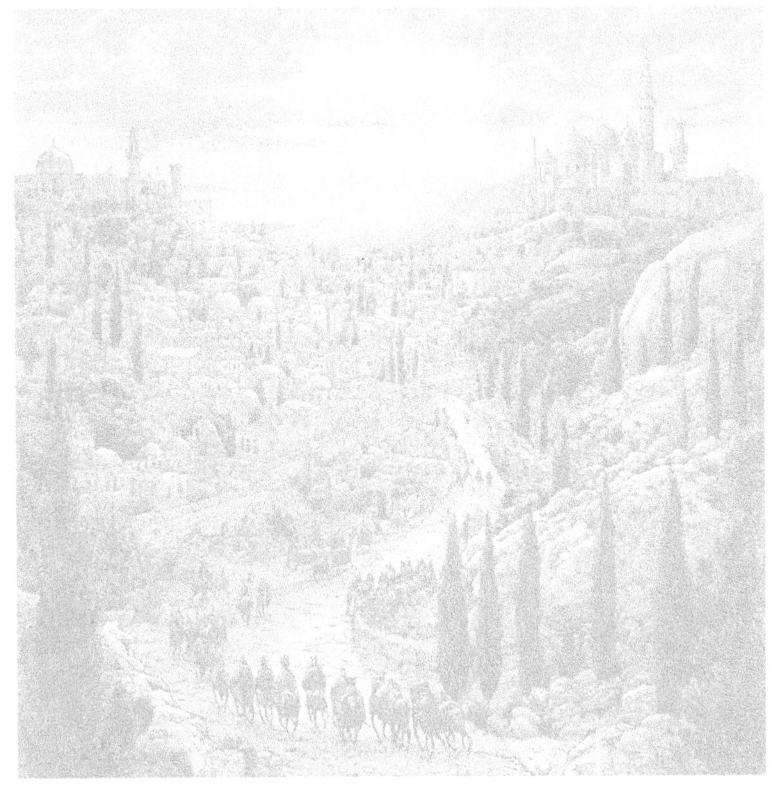

There are six prominent *moadim* ["appointed times"] that are celebrated: *Rosh Hashanah* ["head of the year"], Yom Kippur ["Day of Atonement"]. *Pesach* ["Passover"], *HaSefirot HaOmer* ["Counting of the Omer"], *Shav'uot* ["Pentecost"], and *Sukkot* ["Booths" or "Tabernacles"]. Of these six, the three pilgrimage festivals (*Pesach*, *Shavuot*, *Sukkot*) serve to highlight our relationship with God. The number three also represents *completeness* and *stability*. For example:

- *The three-fold personhood of God: Father, Son, and Holy Spirit.*
- *Noah had three sons: Shem, Ham, and Japheth.*
- *There were three patriarchs of Israel: Abraham, Isaac, and Jacob.*
- *The Ark of the Covenant held three objects: a golden jar of manna, Aaron's budded staff, and the tablets containing the Ten Commandments.*
- *Daniel prayed three times a day.*
- *The prophet Jonah was in the belly of the great fish for three days.*
- *According to the Torah, men were required to present themselves at the Temple three times a year (Feasts of Unleavened Bread, Weeks, and Tabernacles).*
- *Yeshua was tempted by the Adversary three times in the wilderness.*
- *Peter denied knowing Yeshua three times.*
- *Yeshua was in the grave for three days.*

The life of Yeshua fulfilled the old covenant, and his death, burial, and resurrection formed a new covenant into which everyone is now invited. However, if we are to experience the fullness of this new covenant, we must strive to live in harmonious balance between the Law and the Spirit.

The purpose of the Law was to illustrate our need for a Savior...

ROMANS 10:4 CJB | [4] For the goal at which the Torah [Law] aims is the Messiah, who offers righteousness to everyone who trusts.

And Yeshua himself spoke to the importance of honoring the Law...

MATTHEW 5:17-19 CJB | [17] "Don't think that I [Yeshua] have come to abolish the Torah [Law] or the Prophets. I have come not to abolish but to complete.
[18] Yes indeed! I tell you that until heaven and earth pass away, not so much as a yud or a stroke will pass from the Torah — not until everything that must happen has happened. [19] So whoever disobeys the least of these mitzvot [commands] and teaches others to do so will be called the least in the Kingdom of Heaven. But whoever obeys them and so teaches will be called great in the Kingdom of Heaven.

But Yeshua also offers us freedom to live in him while still honoring the Law.

GALATIANS 2:14-16 CJB | [14] [...] I [Paul] said to Kefa [Peter], right in front of everyone, "If you, who are a Jew, live like a Goy [Gentile] and not like a Jew, why are you forcing the Goyim [Gentiles] to live like Jews? [15] We are Jews by birth, not so-called 'Goyishe sinners'; [16] even so, we have come to realize that a person is not declared righteous by God on the ground of his legalistic observance of Torah commands, but through the Messiah Yeshua's [Jesus] trusting faithfulness.

Since Yeshua already fulfilled the Law, we now celebrate these festivals with him...as Lord, as Savior, as friend, as co-heirs in his kingdom. Whereas the observances previously required by the Law were a matter of righteousness, now our righteousness is found in *him*. Therefore, the *only* reason we celebrate these *moadim* ["appointed time(s)"] is to draw closer to our *Abba* ["Dear Father"]. For example, God instructed the Israelites how to celebrate *Pesach* [Passover]...

EXODUS 12:1-11 CJB | [1] ADONAI spoke to Moshe [Moses] and Aharon [Aaron] in the land of Egypt; he said, [2] "You are to begin your calendar with this month; it will be the first month of the year for you.

JOSHUA 5:10-12 CJB | 10 The people of Isra'el camped at Gilgal, and they observed Pesach [Passover] on the fourteenth day of the month, there on the plains of Yericho [Jericho]. 11 The day after Pesach they ate what the land produced, matzah [unleavened bread] and roasted ears of grain that day. 12 The following day, after they had eaten food produced in the land, the man [mana] ended. From then on, the people of Isra'el no longer had man; instead, that year, they ate the produce of the land of Kena'an [Canaan].

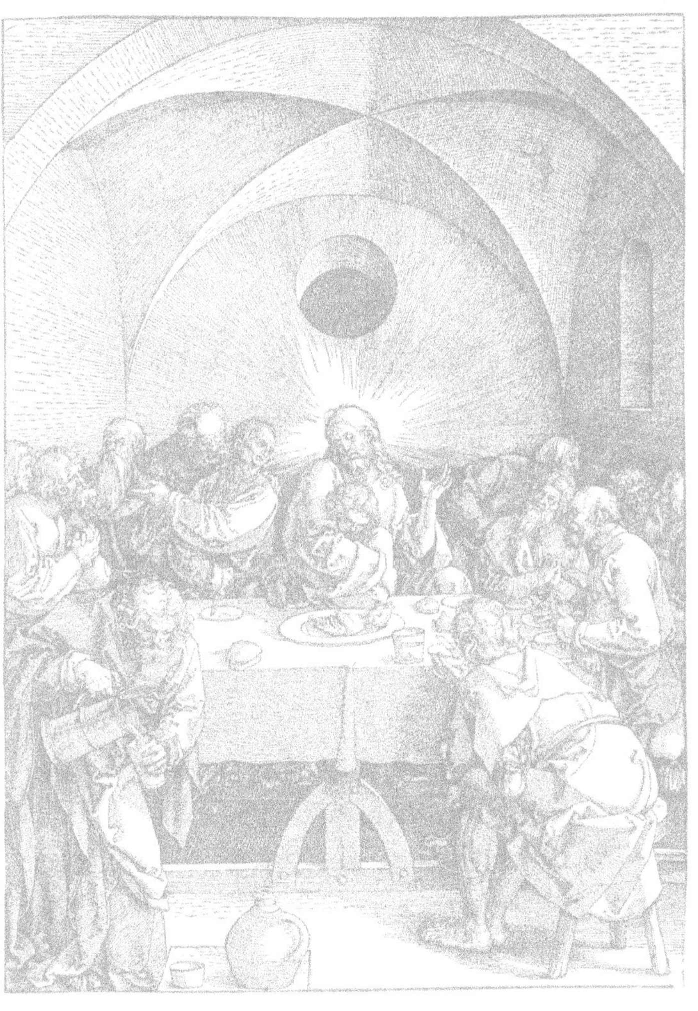

And also, Yeshua's followers...

LUKE 22:1, 7-8, 17-20 CJB | 1 But the festival of Matzah [Unleavened Bread], known as Pesach [Passover], was approaching; [...]

7 Then came the day of matzah [unleavened bread], on which the Passover lamb had to be killed. 8 Yeshua [Jesus] sent Kefa [Peter] and Yochanan [John], instructing them, "Go and prepare our Seder [ceremonial dinner], so we can eat." [...]

17 Then, taking a cup of wine, he [Jesus] made the b'rakhah [blessing] and said, "Take this and share it among yourselves. 18 For I tell you that from now on, I will not drink the 'fruit of the vine' until the Kingdom of God comes."

19 Also, taking a piece of matzah, he made the b'rakhah, broke it, gave it to them and said, "This is my body, which is being given for you; do this in memory of me." 20 He did the same with the cup after the meal, saying, "This cup is the New Covenant, ratified by my blood, which is being poured out for you."

> **1 CORINTHIANS 5:7-8 CJB** | [7] [...] For our Pesach [Passover] lamb, the Messiah, has been sacrificed. [8] So let us celebrate the Seder not with leftover hametz [yeast], the hametz of wickedness and evil, but with the matzah [unleavened bread] of purity and truth.

Why Did Christians Stop Celebrating The Festivals?

As previously noted, [see **PART 2: A Forgotten History, pp. 69-86**] the Church has a complicated relationship with its Hebrew roots so its hardly surprising there is considerable confusion surrounding how (or even if) followers of Yeshua should celebrate the festivals. For this reason, Jewish and Christian leaders, both historically and in the present day, have often objected to Gentile observances of *Pesach* [Passover] et al. However, these objections are almost exclusively founded upon the *"ecclesiastical anti-Judaism that developed after the Church's first century."*

It should be remembered that before welcoming Gentiles into the Council of Jerusalem (c. 50 AD), the vast majority of its communicants were Jews; therefore, the observation of Passover was naturally expected.

> *"Its celebration represented a significant part of the biblical heritage upon which the early Jewish leaders of the Church had founded a faith that recognized Yeshua [Jesus] as the fulfillment of the Messianic prophecies and as the Savior of the world."*

As time passed, Gentiles (and their traditions) gradually assumed greater places of prominence within the Church which only intensified socio-political pressure to disassociate themselves from "all things Jewish." Emperor Constantine's legalization of Christianity and the Nicaean Creed subsequently completed this separation of the Hebrew roots from the Christian faith.

There was also a great deal of controversy raging over whether absolute obedience to Mosaic Law was essential for salvation...*in addition to faith in Yeshua*. Of particular concern was the practice of circumcision. Specifically, the question of whether it should be required of new converts to Judeo-Christianity...or if the "circumcision of the heart" that God had described to

Moses, Jeremiah, and Paul was sufficient *without* the physical procedure.

In some of his letters, Paul openly criticized that particular segment of the Jewish community (both in traditional Judaism and in the Messianic community) who believed salvation was the reward for submission to, and ritual observance of, God's law. Unfortunately, this social criticism between fellow Jews was misunderstood and erroneously generalized by later Gentile church leaders.

Rather than embrace Paul's balanced position on the interrelationship between faith in Yeshua and the Law, later church leaders simply insisted that Christians shared nothing in common with Jews and Judaism.

This position was especially evident in relation to the ecclesiastical holy days that were changed from their original 1st century practice to accommodate the various cultures and pagan religions into which the Christian faith had expanded.

For instance, *Shabbat* ["Sabbath"] was moved from Saturday to Sunday—a day devoted to worship Mithra, the sun god. Passages such as Colossians 2:16-17 were quoted to convince Christians that all "Jewish" holy days and Sabbaths had been somehow abandoned by the Church.

> **COLOSSIANS 2:16-17 CJB** | [16] So don't let anyone pass judgment on you in connection with eating and drinking, or in regard to a Jewish festival or Rosh-Chodesh [first fruits] or Shabbat [Sabbath]. [17] These are a shadow of things that are coming, but the body is of the Messiah.

Additionally, virtually all of Christendom—including the reform movements that began in the 16th century and continuing afterward—fully embraced a supercessionist view toward Jews and Judaism. This view asserted that:

1. **Christianity had forever replaced Judaism in God's plan for salvation.**

2. **Christians had forever replaced the Jews as God's chosen people, who were cursed because they rejected Yeshua (Jesus) as their Messiah.**

Ripped from its Hebrew moorings, Christianity was suddenly cast adrift on the tides of various humanistic worldviews that enabled the persecution of Jews. *Is it any wonder then, that it became unthinkable for Christians to celebrate the "Jewish" festivals? Even today, much of the Western Church remains wary of any involvement in "Jewish" practices.*

Thankfully, growing numbers of Christians are rejecting these historically indefensible arguments, rediscovering the Hebraic roots of Christianity, and asking a very simple question, *"If it was right for Jesus and his apostles, then why isn't it right for me?"*

These teachings and practices were clearly an important aspect of the Messianic community's system of praise, worship, and service during the 1st century. And through this reconnection with our "New/Old Testament" heritage, God is inviting us to experience a deeper, richer relationship with Him.

It is important for both Jews and Christians alike to recognize that the Gentile understanding of prophecies and practices in the Hebrew Scriptures rests on interpretations of those Scriptures by *1st century Jews who viewed Yeshua of Nazareth as the promised Messiah*.

Yeshua himself was a *Torah*-observant Jew. All the apostles upon whom the Messianic community was established were *Torah*-observant Jews. During the first decade following Yeshua's resurrection, almost every member of the Messianic Community was a *Torah*-observant Jew. Indeed, many of their number were even Pharisees (Acts 15:5) and Temple priests (Acts 6:7).

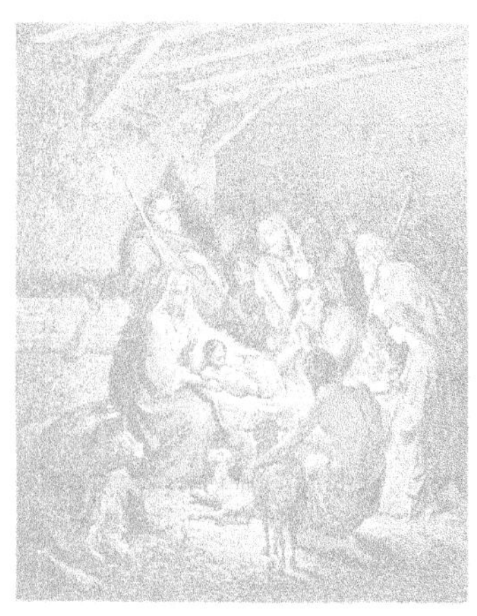

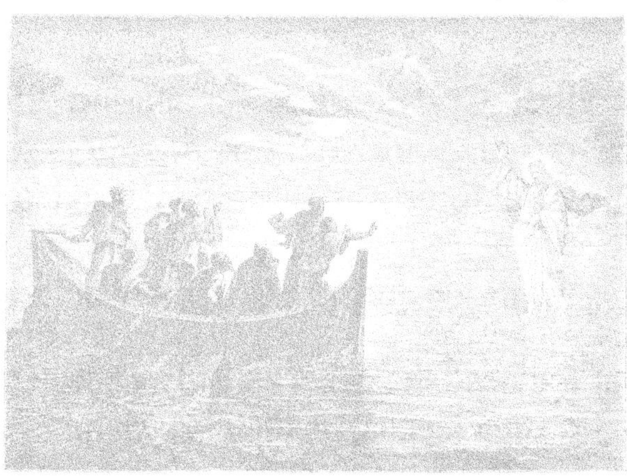

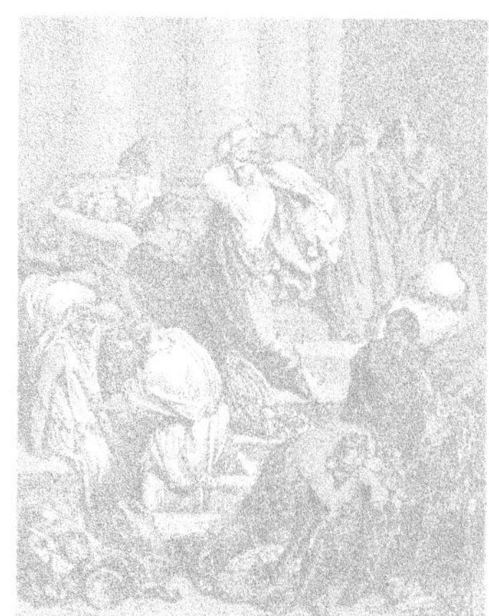

Since no single branch of Judaism was dominant at that time, Messianic Jews were not obligated to interpret Scripture according to the overarching dogmas or theological systems embraced by members of the traditional Jewish community (e.g., Pharisees, Sadducees, Temple priests, etc.).

Therefore, Messianic interpretations of the festivals that find their fulfillment in Yeshua have been reliably established on *Jewish* interpretation.

In other words, *Jewish followers of Yeshua celebrated the various festival traditions of their day and infused them with additional meaning from the life, death, resurrection, and ascension of Yeshua.*

For example, early Jewish leaders of the Messianic community interpreted the Passover events as an allegory that pointed to Yeshua. The Gentile Christians' later allegorical interpretations of the Exodus/Passover events merely expanded upon this foundation laid by their Jewish predecessors. But the seeds of these beliefs originated in the fertile hearts of observant *Jews*... Yeshua and his apostles.

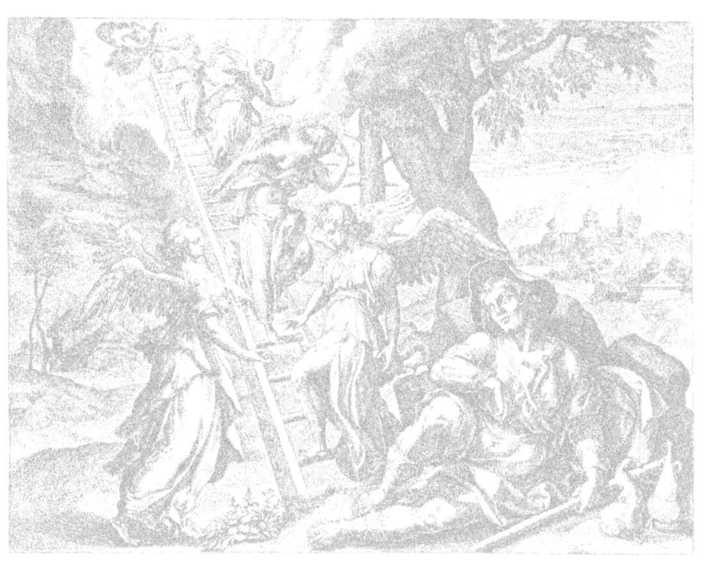

Consequently, these ideas are absolutely authentic *Jewish interpretations*, not Gentile utterances that can be casually dismissed as lacking legitimacy.

The Hebrew Scriptures foretold that the Jews would open the door of faith to Gentiles, predicting that "Israel's light would be carried to the Nations of the world."

ISAIAH 42:6 CJB | 6 "I, ADONAI, called you [Israel] righteously, I took hold of you by the hand, I shaped you and made you a covenant for the people, to be a light for the Goyim [Gentiles] 7 so that you can open blind eyes, free the prisoners from confinement, those living in darkness from the dungeon.

ISAIAH 49:6 CJB | [6] [God] has said, "It is not enough that you are merely my servant to raise up the tribes of Ya'akov [Jacob] and restore the offspring of Isra'el. I will also make you [Israel] a light to the nations, so my salvation can spread to the ends of the earth."

LUKE 2:30-32 CJB | [30] for I [Simon] have seen with my own eyes your yeshu'ah [salvation], [31] which you prepared in the presence of all peoples—[32] a light that will bring revelation to the Goyim [Gentiles] and glory to your people Isra'el."

ACTS 13:47 CJB | [47] For that is what ADONAI has ordered us [Jews] to do: "I have set you as a light for the Goyim [Gentiles], to be for deliverance to the ends of the earth."

These Scriptures explain why every Gentile added to Messianic Community (i.e., the body of Yeshua) becomes united with the Jews in every way... spiritually, relationally, and even nationally.

EPHESIANS 2:11-16 CJB | [11] Therefore, remember your former state: you Gentiles by birth — called the Uncircumcised by those who, merely because of an operation on their flesh, are called the Circumcised —[12] at that time had no Messiah. You were estranged from the national life of Isra'el. You were foreigners to the covenants embodying God's promise. You were in this world without hope and without God.

[13] But now, you who were once far off have been brought near through the shedding of the Messiah's blood. [14] For he himself is our shalom [peace] — he has made us both one and has broken down the m'chitzah [separating wall] which divided us [15] by destroying in his own body the enmity occasioned by the Torah [the Law], with its commands set forth in the form of ordinances.

He did this in order to create in union with himself from the two groups a single new humanity and thus make shalom, [16] and in order to reconcile to God both in a single body by being executed on a stake as a criminal and thus in himself killing that enmity.

Ultimately, every Gentile follower of Yeshua was considered by their Jewish brethren to have been grafted into God's family tree of salvation and covenant relationship (the theme of Romans 11).

FAITH

Even in ancient Israel, a proselyte was acknowledged as though he had been born to Jewish parents.

Coupled with Paul's declaration to Gentile believers (Romans 4:12,16) that Abraham was "the father of us all [Jew and Gentile]," the apostle clearly regarded Gentiles who trusted in the Messiah as children of the patriarch, Abraham.

With this in mind, it is only natural for followers of Yeshua to long to rediscover the roots of their faith and to find their way back home. Although Gentiles by birth, we have been added to the Nation of Israel through faith in Yeshua. As fellow citizens with the saints of Israel, we are entitled to share in the heritage of God's chosen people.

For example, if one were to immigrate to another nation of the modern world, they could (1) remain a foreigner or (2) enter the process of naturalization. In the United States when one takes the Oath of Allegiance, they become *just as much a citizen* as the person whose ancestors signed the Declaration of Independence...and they *share the same rights*.

Pesach [Passover] serves as a perfect illustration. This festival celebrates Israel's liberation from Egyptian slavery...which set them on the path toward Mount Sinai to enter a covenant with God as His Chosen Nation of Priests.

Thus, this event is foundational to both Judaism and Christianity, because without Passover...there would be no nation of Israel for Yeshua to descend from...and there would be no Yeshua into whom Gentile believers could be added as "naturalized" citizens of Israel.

Pesach [Passover] At A Glance...

Traditional Celebration: *Pesach* commemorates when God delivered the Israelites from 430 years of slavery in Egypt (Exodus 12:40-41). It begins with the *Seder* meal on the first night, where foods like *matzah* ["unleavened bread"], *maror* ["bitter herbs"], and a roasted lamb shank are served to symbolize different aspects of the Exodus. Additionally, (1) the *Haggadah* (a Jewish text that describes the order of the *Seder*) is recited to retell the story of God's deliverance and (2) no leavened bread is consumed for seven days in remembrance of the haste with which Israel departed Egypt.

Historical Significance: *Pesach* marks the defining moment in Hebrew history when God delivered His people from slavery in Egypt through the tenth plague, when the firstborn of Egypt was struck down. This singular event is central to the covenant relationship between God and Israel, as it led to (1) liberation from their oppressors and (2) the journey to enter to the Promised Land.

Spiritual Significance: *Pesach* illustrates God's power to redeem His people and to liberate them from both physical and spiritual bondage. It is a *Moadim* ["appointed time"] to reflect on God's mighty works, His faithfulness to His promises, and the call for His people to live in obedience and purity.

Messianic Meaning: For the Messianic community, *Pesach* takes on additional meaning as we view Yeshua (Jesus) as the Passover Lamb (John 1:29), who was sacrificed to bring redemption to all of humanity. The parallels between the blood of the lambs in Egypt that protected Israel from death and the blood of Yeshua's sacrificial death on the cross highlight the Messianic fulfillment of this festival. The breaking of *matzah* ["unleavened bread"] and drinking of wine during the *Seder* point to Yeshua's final *Seder* with his disciples before his atoning death on the cross.

A Deeper Look At Pesach [Passover]

Should Christians celebrate Passover? This is a legitimate question, and we must seek the answer in Scripture, not religious opinion.

> **1 CORINTHIANS 5:7-8 CJB** | [7] Get rid of the old hametz [yeast], so that you can be a new batch of dough, because in reality you are unleavened. For our Pesach [Passover] lamb, the Messiah, has been sacrificed. [8] So let us celebrate the Seder not with leftover hametz, the hametz of wickedness and evil, but with the matzah [unleavened bread] of purity and truth.

Think about that for a moment. A *Jewish* apostle issued this directive to *Gentiles*.

How Should Christians Observe The Passover?

Naturally, the best answer comes from Jesus himself. According to the Gospels, he celebrated the Passover with his disciples with a traditional *Seder* meal (but our freedom in the Messiah permits great flexibility of practice).

To avoid any possible confusion on the matter, Paul offers liturgical instruction for remembering the Messiah's sacrificial death in the Passover celebration:

> **1 CORINTHIANS 11:23-26 CJB** | [23] For what I received from the Lord is just what I passed on to you — that the Lord Yeshua [Jesus], on the night he was betrayed, took bread; [24] and after he had made the b'rakhah [blessing] he broke it and said, "This is my body, which is for you. Do this as a memorial to me"; [25] likewise also the cup after the meal, saying, "This cup is the New Covenant effected by my blood; do this, as often as you drink it, as a memorial to me."
>
> [26] For as often as you eat this bread and drink the cup, you proclaim the death of the Lord, until he comes.

On the same night, thousands of years earlier, lambs were sacrificed to protect the homes of the Hebrews from the plague of death…hours before

Moses would lead them out of slavery in Egypt. Likewise, Yeshua, the Lamb of God, would be sacrificed to complete the law and save both Jew and Gentile from the slavery of sin and death.

The blood of Jesus saves, frees, and heals us. But the depth of this profound moment is incomplete without understanding all that happened on this historic date. We are gifted the opportunity to personally experience, as sons and daughters, the fulfillment of God's promise granting partnership in the covenant of Abraham and the full citizenship of Heaven.

Sefirat HaOmer ["Counting the Omer"] At A Glance...

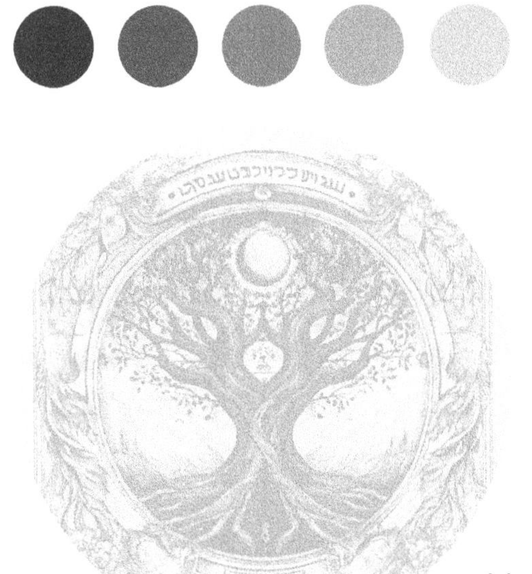

Traditional Celebration: *Sefirat HaOmer* is the 49-day period between *Pesach* and *Shavuot*. Each day is counted with a blessing, starting from the second day of *Pesach*, to prepare for the arrival of *Shavuot*. This period is a time spiritual anticipation and reflection, often considered a time of personal growth and preparation.

Historical Significance: Traditionally, the *Omer* was a sheaf of barley offered in the Temple on the second day of *Pesach*, marking the beginning of the grain harvest. Thus, the *Sefirat HaOmer* linked the physical harvest cycle to the spiritual anticipation of receiving the *Torah* on *Shavuot*.

Spiritual Significance: The *Sefirat HaOmer* symbolizes spiritual progress and training, as the Israelites prepared to meet God at Mount Sinai. It is a reminder of the importance of discipline and anticipation in the life of faith.

Messianic Meaning: The Messianic community sees the *Sefirat HaOmer* as a time of anticipation of the Holy Spirit which culminated in *Shavuot* [Pentecost]. Just as the disciples waited for the promised Holy Spirit during this time, we now reflect on the fullness of God's revelation through His Word and His Spirit.

A Deeper Look At Sefirat HaOmer ["Counting the Omer"]

Although this is probably the least well-known Jewish celebration among modern followers of Jesus, the instructions concerning the counting...

> **LEVITICUS 23:15-16 CJB** | 15 "'From the day after the day of rest [Sabbath]— that
> is, from the day you bring the sheaf for waving — you are to count seven full
> weeks, 16 until the day after the seventh week; you are to count fifty days; and
> then you are to present a new grain offering to ADONAI.

...actually foreshadowed the second coming of the Messiah.

> **1 CORINTHIANS 15:20-23 CJB** | [20] But the fact is that the Messiah has been raised from the dead, the *firstfruits* of those who have died. [21] For since death came through a man, also the resurrection of the dead has come through a man. [22] For just as in connection with Adam all die, so in connection with the Messiah all will be made alive. [23] But each in his own order: the Messiah is the *firstfruits*; then those who belong to the Messiah, at the time of his coming;

An *omer* generally refers to one-tenth of a bushel dry-measure of grain. According to the *Torah*, an *omer* of new grain must be waived before the altar on each of the 49 days between *Pesach* and *Shav'uot*.

This is called "waving the *Omer*" and prior to offering this new grain (or first-fruits), only produce from earlier harvests is permitted to be eaten. In other words, only crops that have first been dedicated to God are considered *kosher* (acceptable) and this is why they are considered a "first-fruits" offering.

Israel was instructed by the *Torah* [Law] to count 49 days (i.e., seven weeks of days) from *Pesach* [Passover] until *Shav'uot* [Pentecost].

This period of counting is called *Sephirot HaOmer* ["counting of the sheaves"]. A blessing is spoken over each day declaring exactly how many more days are left before the seven weeks of days are complete. For this reason, Psalm 67 is often recited because it's composed of 49 Hebrew words which correspond to the 49 days of the *Omer* count.

> **PSALM 67:1-8 CJB** | [1] For the leader. With stringed instruments. A psalm. A song: [2] God, be gracious to us, and bless us. May he make his face shine toward us, (Selah "to praise.") [3] so that your way may be known on earth, your salvation among all nations. [4] Let the peoples give thanks to you, God; let the peoples give thanks to you, all of them. [5] Let the nations be glad and shout for joy, for you will judge the peoples fairly and guide the nations on earth. (Selah) [6] Let the peoples give thanks to you, God; let the peoples give thanks to you, all of them. [7] The earth has yielded its harvest; may God, our God, bless us. [8] May God continue to bless us, so that all the ends of the earth will fear him.

The Hebrew Meaning Of The Counting

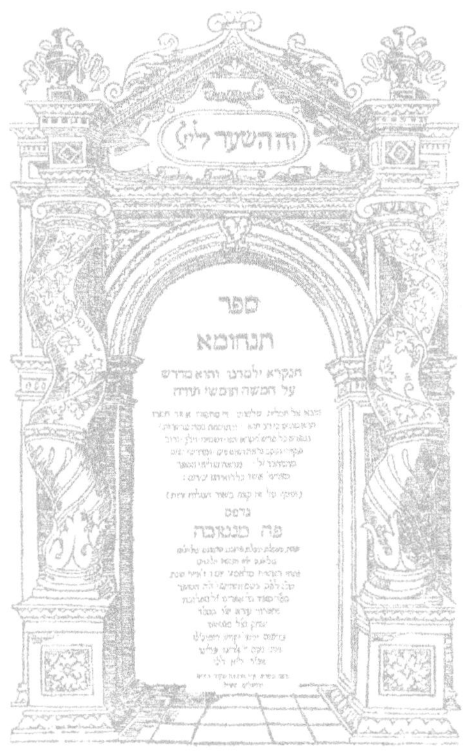

According to the *Midrash*, a genre of rabbinic literature containing Jewish textual interpretations and compilations of homilies, it was foretold that they would receive the *Torah* exactly 50 days after their exodus from Egypt. It was said that the Hebrews were so eager to receive this revelation that after being delivered from Egypt, they immediately began counting the days. Thus, the counting of days from *Pesach* to *Shav'uot* also commemorates their eagerness to receive the *Torah*.

After reciting the Psalm 67 blessing, the count of the *Omer* is traditionally declared in both days and weeks. For example, on the first day they would say, "Today is day one of the *Omer*", etc. Then, on the eighth day they would say, "Today is is eight days, which is one week and one day of the *Omer*." This continues day by day until the 49th day when they would say, "Today is 49 days, which are seven weeks of the *Omer*."

The counting is performed this way because the Jewish sages interpret "you shall count for yourselves" to mean that one should count each day of the *Omer* aloud, usually at the conclusion of the daily evening prayer service.

The celebration of *Pesach* culminates in *Shav'uot* when we remember Israel's (and ours) deliverance through the revelation of the *Torah*. During the time between, we are called to sanctify ourselves for personal revelation by engaging in seven weeks of repentance. That is why the blessing is recited each day in anticipation of *Shav'uot*.

As previously noted, the *Omer* ends after counting seven weeks, or 7 x 7 days from *Pesach* to *Shav'uot*, with the symmetry of the counting suggesting both perfection and completion.

According to the Jewish sages, the first revelation was given at Mount Sinai, and then greater revelation was given at Zion. This is why they believe the redemption process began at *Pesach* and was completed at *Shav'uot*.

In later Jewish tradition, the 49 days between *Pesach* and *Shav'uot* marked the time between the festival of physical redemption (*Pesach*) and the festival of spiritual redemption (*Shav'uot*). The connection between these two festivals beautifully illustrate how the righteousness required by the Law was fulfilled in Yeshua and is available to all who trust him.

> **ROMANS 10:4 CJB** | [4] For the goal at which the Torah [the Law] aims is the Messiah, who offers righteousness to everyone who trusts.

Shav'uot commemorates two important events in human history: First, God's giving of the *Torah* (Old Covenant) to Israel at Mount Sinai and second, the giving of the Holy Spirit (New Covenant) to both Jew and Gentile.

The first covenant (based on Mosaic law) was fulfilled in the second through our deliverance in Yeshua, the True Lamb of God, and then confirmed by the Holy Spirit.

Perhaps it was with a touch of divine irony that during the season when Jews from around the world pilgrimage to Jerusalem to reaffirm their commitment to the Mosaic covenant, the Holy Spirit descended upon Jews from every nation to offer the new covenant to all who would believe (Acts 2:1-42).

> **JEREMIAH 31:32-33 CJB** | [32] "For this is the covenant I will make with the house of Isra'el after those days," says ADONAI: "I will put my Torah within them and write it on their hearts; I will be their God, and they will be my people. [33] No longer will any of them teach his fellow community member or his brother, 'Know ADONAI'; for all will know me, from the least of them to the greatest; because I will forgive their wickednesses and remember their sins no more."

This new covenant fulfills the old by inscribing the *Torah* on our hearts instead of on stone tablets. The Holy Spirit now guides us into all wisdom and understanding as we experience a life fruitful in the liberty given to us through the love and grace of our Lord Yeshua.

HEBREWS 10:16-17 CJB | [16] "'This is the covenant which I will make with them after those days,' says ADONAI: 'I will put my Torah [Law] on their hearts, and write it on their minds...'"

[17] he then adds, "'And their sins and their wickednesses I will remember no more.'"

Should Followers Of Yeshua Count The Omer?

The reason for counting the *Omer* was to foretell the giving of the Holy Spirit and to confirm God's new covenant. The redemption process set in motion at *Pesach* was completed at *Shav'uot*, and that completion revealed God's love through His offer of deliverance, in Yeshua, for the whole world.

Prophetically, the "first-fruits" celebration of the waving of the *Omer* prefigures Jew and Gentile being formed into a "single new humanity"...in union with Yeshua to worship God.

EPHESIANS 2:11-16 CJB | [11] Therefore, remember your former state: you Gentiles by birth — called the Uncircumcised by those who, merely because of an operation on their flesh, are called the Circumcised — [12] at that time had no Messiah. You were estranged from the national life of Isra'el. You were foreigners to the covenants embodying God's promise. You were in this world without hope and without God.

[13] But now, you who were once far off have been brought near through the shedding of the Messiah's blood. [14] For he himself is our shalom — he has made us both one and has broken down the m'chitzah [middle wall of the boundary fence] which divided us [15] by destroying in his own body the enmity occasioned by the Torah [Law], with its commands set forth in the form of ordinances.

He did this in order to create in union with himself from the two groups a single new humanity and thus make shalom [peace], [16] and in order to reconcile to God both in a single body by being executed on a stake as a criminal and thus in himself killing that enmity.

The countdown to *Shav'uot* extends beyond the revelation of *Torah* given at Sinai and points to the greater revelation at Zion. Yeshua removed our sin and became our righteousness through his sacrifice as the true Passover Lamb upon the cross. Thus, *Shav'uot* is the fulfillment of the promise of the Holy Spirit to those who trust in Him.

How Should Followers Of Yeshua Count The Omer?

As members of the Messianic Community, we recognize the Jewish traditions of our faith and embrace the relational meaning behind these set apart times on God's calendar. However, since we have full freedom in Yeshua, *it's simply a matter of how you would like to honor this time and season.*

For example, in our home, we count down the days and pray around sundown, sometimes together, sometimes on our own. We sometimes read the Bible or devotional books and journal to help us explore deeper areas of our hearts that need repentance. As a family, we enjoy celebrating *Shav'uot* with a meal and *challah* bread (especially since we couldn't have any at *Pesach*)! ☺

Because of the resurrection and its connection to *Shav'uot* [Pentecost], the counting of the *Omer* is a symbolic and deeply enriching experience for believers. It is interesting to note that all of Yeshua's appearances following his resurrection occurred within the 49 days of the *Omer* count. Some of these appearances were as follows:

Nissan 18 [April 8]

Mary Magdalene had seven demons cast out of her during the first part of Yeshua's ministry (Mark 16:9; Luke 8:2-3) and later became part of his inner circle of close family and friends. She was the first person Yeshua revealed himself to after his resurrection (Mark 16:9-11; John 20:11-18).

Two men were walking to Emmaus, a small village roughly seven miles from Jerusalem, when Yeshua revealed himself to them (Luke 24:13-33). He gently chided them for not believing what the prophets foretold regarding the Messiah and then explained all the Scripture that pertained to himself.

It was not until sitting down together for a meal that the two men had "their eyes opened" and recognized Yeshua before he vanished from their sight!

Nissan 19 [April 9]

For the first time, Yeshua revealed himself to the disciples who had attended his last *Pesach* meal. For reasons unknown, Thomas was not in attendance. (John 20:19).

Following Yeshua's departure, the disciples informed Thomas of the visitation.

> **JOHN 20:25 CJB** | 25 When the other talmidim [disciples] told him [Thomas], "We have seen the Lord," he replied, "Unless I see the nail marks in his hands, put my finger into the place where the nails were and put my hand into his side, I refuse to believe it."

Nissan 26 [April 16]

Yeshua again revealed himself to his disciples, but this time Thomas was present, and it marked the first time that all his disciples (excepting Judas) with whom he shared *Pesach*, saw him together.

Yeshua allowed Thomas to observe and touch the wounds he received in order to strengthen his faith.

> **JOHN 20:26-29 CJB** | 26 A week later his talmidim [disciples] were once more in the room, and this time T'oma [Thomas] was with them. Although the doors were locked, Yeshua [Jesus] came, stood among them and said, "Shalom aleikhem!" ["peace be upon you"] 27
>
> Then he said to T'oma, "Put your finger here, look at my hands, take your hand and put it into my side. Don't be lacking in trust but have trust!" 28
>
> T'oma answered him, "My Lord and my God!" 29
>
> Yeshua said to him, "Have you trusted because you have seen me? How blessed are those who do not see but trust anyway!"

Nissan 27 to Iyyar 26 [April 17 to May 17]

The apostle Paul was the only New Testament writer to record that following Yeshua's resurrection, he appeared to more than five hundred disciples at one time. However, Paul did not specify an exact date when this event occurred.

> **1 CORINTHIANS 15:6 CJB** | [...] [6] and afterwards he [Yeshua] was seen by more than five hundred brothers at one time, the majority of whom are still alive, though some have died.

After celebrating his final *Pesach*, Yeshua and his eleven disciples (Judas was betraying him then) walked toward the Garden of Gethsemane and he said, "But after I have been raised, I will go ahead of you into the Galil [Galilee]." (Matthew 26:32; Mark 14:28 CJB). The book of Matthew records this meeting.

> **MATTHEW 28:16-18 CJB** | [16] So the eleven talmidim [disciples] went to the hill in the Galil [Galilee] where Yeshua had told them to go. [17] When they saw him, they prostrated themselves before him; but some hesitated. [18] Yeshua came and talked with them. [...]

Yeshua revealed himself to seven of his disciples while they were fishing on Lake Galilee (John 21:1-24). Those disciples were Peter, John, James, Thomas, Nathanael, and two other unnamed disciples (likely Andrew and Philip, who resided in the general area).

Peter miraculously caught 153 fish in his net and Yeshua asked him three times if he loved him. It was at that time that Peter learned he would die a martyrs' death and Yeshua implied that John would live long enough to write about his Second Coming at the end of the age.

Yeshua made a special appearance to James, his physical half-brother (Matthew 13:55; Mark 6:3; Galatians 1:19). According to Paul, this occurred between Yeshua's appearance before 500+ people and his appearance to all the apostles (1 Corinthians 15:5-7). However, it is unclear whether Paul is referring to Yeshua's first meeting in Galilee or his final appearance when he ascended into heaven.

Iyyar 27 [May 18]

When Yeshua met with his disciples on the Mount of Olives (Acts 1) just prior to his ascension, he gave them the "Great Commission" and instructions to wait ten more days in the city of Jerusalem to receive the power of the Holy Spirit (Matthew 28:18-20; Mark 16:15-18; Acts 1:4-9).

ACTS 1:4-11 CJB | 4 At one of these gatherings, he instructed them not to leave Yerushalayim [Jerusalem] but to wait for "what the Father promised, which you heard about from me. 5 For Yochanan [John] used to immerse people in water; but in a few days, you will be immersed in the Ruach HaKodesh [Holy Spirit]!"

6 When they were together, they asked him, "Lord, are you at this time going to restore self-rule to Isra'el?" 7 He answered, "You don't need to know the dates or the times; the Father has kept these under his own authority. 8 But you will receive power when the Ruach HaKodesh comes upon you; you will be my witnesses both in Yerushalayim and in all Y'hudah [Judea] and Shomron [Samaria], indeed to the ends of the earth!"

9 After saying this, he was taken up before their eyes; and a cloud hid him from their sight. 10 As they were staring into the sky after him, suddenly they saw two men dressed in white standing next to them. 11 The men said, "You Galileans! Why are you standing, staring into space? This Yeshua, who has been taken away from you into heaven, will come back to you in just the same way as you saw him go into heaven."

Sivan 8 [May 28]

The disciples obeyed Yeshua's instructions to wait ten days in Jerusalem and on *Shav'uot* God gave His Spirit to more than 3,120 people (Acts 2)! After his resurrection, Yeshua's ministry established the groundwork for launching his Messianic Community.

As the blood of the lamb represented Israel's deliverance and the giving of the *Torah* at Mount Sinai (old covenant)...so the death of Yeshua on the cross represented humanity's deliverance and the giving of the Holy Spirit at Jerusalem (new covenant).

And the waving of the loaves (*Omer*) connects these two events together, completing the unification of old and new into Yeshua himself.

> **REVELATION 5:9 CJB** | [9] and they [the 24 elders] sang a new song, "You are worthy to take the scroll and break its seals; because you were slaughtered; at the cost of blood, you ransomed for God persons from every tribe, language, people, and nation. The waving of the two loaves of leavened bread therefore prophesied the creation of the one new man, both Jew and Gentile, that would be first fruits of the Kingdom of God. In the sovereign plan of God Almighty, ultimately there would be one flock and one shepherd for all God's children.

> **JOHN 10:16 CJB** | [16] Also I have other sheep which are not from this pen; I need to bring them, and they will hear my voice; and there will be one flock, one shepherd.

It is interesting to note that the resurrection of Yeshua occurred during the first day of the *Omer* and the Holy Spirit was given to the disciples fifty days later on *Shav'uot*. His ascension was foreshadowed by Moses and the receiving of the *Torah* at Sinai. Just as Moses had waited forty days before Israel received the *Torah*, so the disciples waited forty days before they received the promise of the Holy Spirit.

In both instances, revelation was received at the appointed time...first, in the form of God's voice speaking from the midst of the fire at Mount Sinai, and later, in the form of tongues of fire at Jerusalem speaking the languages of all nations.

A Word About Kabbalah

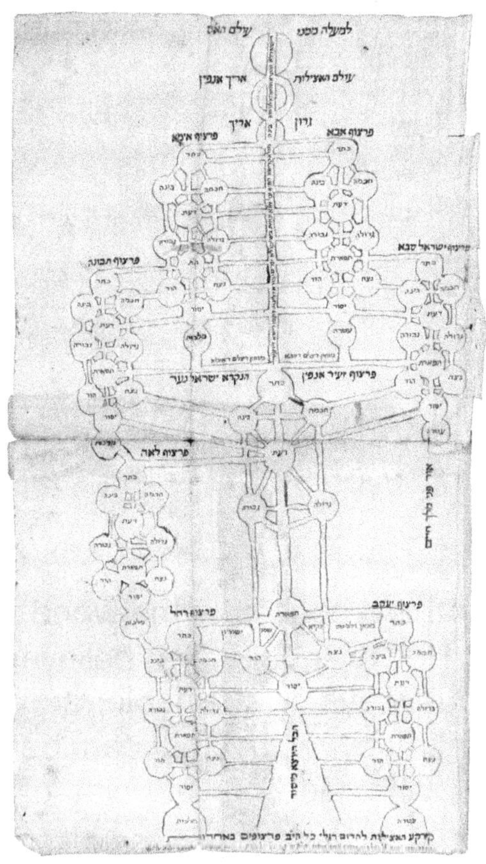

The religion of Kabbalah is based upon the *Zohar* [Heb. "Splendor" or "Radiance"], a collection of mystical commentaries on the *Torah*. Originally written in medieval Aramaic and Hebrew, Kabbalists believe the teachings of the *Zohar* will help them attain greater levels of connectedness with God.

Kabbalah, sometimes translated as "mysticism" or "occult knowledge", is an aspect of Jewish tradition that concerns itself with the "essence of God" and is generally divided into three areas of concentration:

Theoretical
Meditative
Magical

1. The *theoretical*, which concerns itself primarily with the inner dimensions of reality, the spiritual worlds, souls, and angels et. al.

2. The *meditative*, where the goal is to train the student to reach higher meditative states of consciousness and, perhaps, even a prophetical state through employing the divine names, letter permutations, and so forth.

3. The *magical*, which concerns itself with altering and influencing the course of nature using the divine names, incantations, amulets, magical seals, and various other mystical exercises.

These categories are also variously addressed in the books of Deuteronomy and Leviticus:

DEUTERONOMY 18:9-14 CJB | [9] "When you enter the land ADONAI your God is giving you, you are not to learn how to follow the abominable practices of those nations. [10] There must not be found among you anyone who makes his son or daughter pass through fire, a diviner, a soothsayer, an enchanter, a sorcerer, [11] a spell-caster, a consulter of ghosts or spirits, or a necromancer. [12] For whoever does these things is detestable to ADONAI, and because of these abominations ADONAI your God is driving them out ahead of you. [13] You must be wholehearted with ADONAI your God. [14] For these nations, which you are about to dispossess, listen to soothsayers and diviners; but you, ADONAI your God does not allow you to do this.

LEVITICUS 20:6 CJB | [6] "'The person who turns to spirit-mediums and sorcerers to go fornicating after them — I will set myself against him and cut him off from his people.

Whether it involves a sacred text, an experience, or the practices of the world, Kabbalists believe that God's ways are mysterious. However, they also believe full knowledge and understanding of His mysterious ways is attainable, and once equipped with this knowledge, unlimited intimacy with God can be achieved. (Of course, how they define "intimacy with God" is a point of significant divergence from the teachings of Scripture).

As with any false religion, there is *just enough truth to be convincing.*

Practitioners of Kabbalah view the Creator and the Creation as a unified continuum, rather than as distinct entities, and are driven by their desire to experience the "fullness" of God. This desire is intensified by the mystical kinship that Kabbalists believe exists between God and humanity, since within the soul of every individual, is a hidden part of God waiting to be revealed.

But even mystics who reject this supposed "kinship" of God and man, still believe that the entirety of Creation is suffused with divinity. In other words, they reject *all* distinction between "God" and "the universe." Thus, as **Moshe Kordovero (1522-1570)**, a central figure in the historical development of Kabbalah, wrote, "The essence of divinity is found in every single thing, nothing but It exists...It exists in each existent."

Within the three primary concentrations of Kabbalistic teachings previously noted, there are three secondary dimensions of esoteric knowledge common to almost all forms of Jewish mysticism which are likely to be only understood by practitioners who possess specialized knowledge or interest in the topic. Traditionally, this knowledge is believed to be obtainable by:

1. Interpreting sacred texts to uncover *nistar* ["hidden"] meanings.
2. Oral transmission of tradition from a recognized master of Kabbalah.
3. Direct revelation, which could include visitations from angels or Elijah, spirit possession, or some other supra-rational experience.

Unfortunately, the *Omer* has been infected with a great deal of Kabbalist teachings on the subject. For Kabbalists, the 49 days of counting are viewed as a mystical journey through the human soul that returns to Sinai every year.

For this reason, each day of the counting is thought to be associated with one of God's ten *sefirot* ["attributes"]. Kabbalists view these requirements as a multi-layered process of moral and spiritual purification that enables them to experience the exalted heights of the Mount Sinai revelation. They believe that devoting oneself to meditation, repentance, and other activities...ensures their soul 'merits' the gift of re-channeling the universe's divine energy to behold miracles during the 49 days of *teshuva* ["repentance"].

It is interesting to note that Kabbalists regard the 33rd day of the *Omer* count as a "mystic holiday" because it commemorates the date when they claim Kabbalah was revealed to Israel (e.g., as the *Torah* was revealed at Mount Sinai).

According to their sages, each day represents an additional step towards achieving greater clarity of inner meaning. Thus, it is believed that if one mirrors the positive attributes of God, the spark of divine light within our humanity will be *increased.* Conversely, if one indulges laziness or indifference, the spark of divine light within will be *decreased.*

However, contrary to the claims of Kabbalists, Yeshua *never* taught any of these practices to his disciples. Moreover, he taught that humanity was enslaved to sin and in desperate need of deliverance and spiritual rebirth.

Although he preached repentance, Yeshua never suggested human beings were "shattered vessels" who must be reabsorbed into a "Universal Soul."

Moreover, he never taught that God's "hidden essence" was revealed through ten *sefirots* ["attributes"], or that human nature represented a "parallel" to a "sefirotic structure of the universe."

And surely Yeshua would have rejected the Kabbalists' claim that human beings could influence God or His disposition by performing various religious ceremonies or esoteric rituals.

> **MARK 7:5-9 CJB** | 5 The P'rushim [Pharisees] and the Torah-teachers asked him, "Why don't your talmidim [disciples] live in accordance with the Tradition of the Elders, but instead eat with ritually unclean hands?" 6 Yeshua [Jesus] answered them, "Yesha'yahu [Isaiah] was right when he prophesied about you hypocrites — as it is written,
>
> 'These people honor me with their lips, but their hearts are far away from me.
>
> 7 Their worship of me is useless, because they teach man-made rules as if they were doctrines.'
>
> 8 "You depart from God's command and hold onto human tradition. 9 Indeed," he said to them, "you have made a fine art of departing from God's command in order to keep your tradition!"

Moreover, Scriptures teach the supremacy of God as the Creator of all things who has given all authority to the Son who holds everything together.

> **COLOSSIANS 1:14-17 CJB** | 14 It is through his Son that we have redemption — that is, our sins have been forgiven. 15 He is the visible image of the invisible God. He is supreme over all creation, 16 because in connection with him were created all things — in heaven and on earth, visible and invisible, whether thrones, lordships, rulers or authorities — they have all been created through him and for him. 17 He existed before all things, and he holds everything together.

Lastly, Yeshua never taught the idea of *tikken olam* ["repair of the world"] through humanistic self-effort. He plainly taught that HE alone was the Savior of humanity and that our salvation, spiritual life, and the ultimate healing of the world would come solely through him.

> **JOHN 14:6 CJB** | [6] Yeshua said, "I AM the Way — and the Truth and the Life; no one comes to the Father except through me.

This is why we must be so careful of any teaching that elevates self-reliance and self-empowerment above God. It is a spiritual veneer that sounds positive and seems enlightening but instead teaches the deceptive and dangerous idea that "spiritual elevation" and "works righteousness" *are entirely the product of human effort.*

Thus, Kabbalists are fundamentally opposed to the Truth that salvation is found in Yeshua alone. They claim our human nature is essentially an aspect of God and that salvation is simply the process of becoming like Him through the removal of our "outer shell." Clearly, this is not the gospel message that Yeshua preached, nor does it honor his sacrifice as the sole means of obtaining eternal *kapparah* ["atonement"] from God.

In summary, Kabbalah's core concept of *Ein Sof* ["the Infinite"] collapses the biblical distinction between Creator and creation, while *tikkun* teaches that human actions repair fractures within the divine realm itself. Both ideas directly contradict the biblical declaration of a sovereign God who alone initiates and accomplishes redemption.

- God creates (*bara'*, Strong's H1254), He does not emanate.
- God is intrinsically distinct from what He has made (Genesis 1; Isaiah 40; Psalm 33).
- God is not dependent on human action (Psalm 50:12)
- God does not "need repair" (Isaiah 46:9-10)

Since Kabbalah teaches a false system of salvation, it needs to be exposed to members of the Messianic Community who are tempted to dabble in its doctrines, some of which are, at least on the surface, otherwise quite appealing.

Shav'uot [Pentecost] At A Glance

Traditional Celebration: *Shav'uot*, also known as the Feast of Weeks, occurs fifty days after *Pesach* and celebrates the first fruits of the wheat harvest. Traditionally, the Israelites brought their first fruit offerings to the Temple as a sign of gratitude for God's provision. The festival is also associated with the giving of the *Torah* at Mount Sinai, as Jewish tradition holds that this occurred during *Shav'uot*.

Historical Significance: *Shav'uot* marked the transition from the agricultural cycle to one of spiritual focus. It was a time to remember God's provision through the harvest and the great gift of the *Torah*, which provided the Israelites with their laws and guidelines for experiencing an intimate relationship with God.

Spiritual Significance: *Shav'uot* highlights both God's physical provision (through the harvest) and His spiritual provision (through the *Torah*). Thus, it is a celebration of covenant relationship in which God provides not physical and spiritual sustenance as He guides His people into living righteously.

Messianic Meaning: For the Messianic community, *Shav'uot* is also the day of Pentecost, when the Holy Spirit was poured out on the disciples (Acts 2). This event marked the beginning of the new covenant, in which the Holy Spirit writes God's law on the hearts of believers and fulfills the promise of spiritual union (Ezekiel 11:19; Ezekiel 36:26; Jeremiah 31:33; Romans 2:15; Hebrews 8:10). In this way, *Shav'uot* represents the convergence between the giving of the *Torah* and the giving of the Holy Spirit.

A Deeper Look At Shav'uot [Pentecost]

The holiday of *Shav'uot* [Pentecost] is a two-day holiday celebrated from sundown to sundown. The word *Shav'uot* means "weeks" and celebrates the completion of the wheat harvest which symbolizes God's provision. It is marked by the seven-week *Omer* counting period between *Pesach* [Passover] and Shavuot [Pentecost].

Shav'uot is also called, "The Feast of Weeks", or "First Fruits", and represents a foundational moment in Jewish history: the giving of the *Torah* ["Law"] (also called the *Pentateuch*) to the Israelites on Mount Sinai.

The date of celebration falls seven weeks after Passover and commemorates the Hebrews escape from Egyptian slavery when God made them into the nation of Israel. It also means "oaths" and marks when God swore eternal devotion to the Jewish people, who, in return, pledged everlasting loyalty to Him.

In ancient times, two wheat loaves were offered in the Holy Temple on *Shav'uot*. People also brought *bikkurim* ["first fruits"] to thank God for Israel's bounty.

How Is Shav'uot Traditionally Celebrated?

- Women and girls light holiday candles to usher in the holiday, on both the first and second evenings of the holidays.
- It is customary to stay up all night learning *Torah* on the first night of *Shav'uot*.
- All men, women, and children attend synagogue to hear the reading of the Ten Commandments on the first day of *Shav'uot*.
- No "work" may be performed.
- Special traditional meals are eaten, and it is customary to eat dairy foods on *Shav'uot*.
- Some Jews even decorate their homes (and synagogues) with flowers and sweet-smelling plants in advance of *Shav'uot*.

Torah And Prophetic Readings For Shav'uot: Day 1

From the Torah, Exodus 19:1-20:23. This passage recounts the encampment of Israel at the base of Sinai while Moses ascended the mountain to receive God's law and God descended to meet him there.

From the Prophets, Ezekiel 1:1-28. This passage recounts the prophet's ecstatic vision of God's divine chariot. In the same way that Israel nearly caught a glimpse of the divine at Sinai, Ezekiel likewise came close to seeing God in his vision.

Torah And Prophetic Readings For Shav'uot: Day 2

From the Torah, Deuteronomy 14:22-16:17. This passage details the laws for the three pilgrimage festivals: *Pesach* [Passover], *Shav'uot* [Pentecost], and *Sukkot* [Feast of Tabernacles].

From the Prophets, Habakkuk 2:20-3:19. This passage describes the prophet's vision of God, with all the divine hosts, marching to overthrow Israel's enemy—another vision of the divine reminiscent of the encounter at Mount Sinai.

The book of Ruth is also read for three reasons:

1. Ruth (a Moabite) pledged fidelity to Naomi and God mirrors the fidelity that Israel expressed to God upon receiving the *Torah*.

2. Ruth's story takes place during the season of the barley harvest, the agricultural occasion for *Shav'uot*.

3. Ruth is the great-great-grandmother of King David, who is traditionally believed to have been born and died on *Shav'uot*.

Just as God's presence descended on Mount Sinai in fire and sound, the Holy Spirit descended upon the apostles in similar manifestations. In this way, *Shav'uot* is both a reminder of the *Torah's* instructions and a foreshadowing of the Holy Spirit's outpouring on the Day of Pentecost (Acts 2), in fulfilment of God's promise to write His law on believers' hearts rather than on tablets of stone.

The timing and manner of the Holy Spirit's arrival signified a divine transition: the *Torah* written in stone became an internal, transformative reality through the Spirit. This event marked the beginning of the early Messianic Community, empowering believers to spread the gospel through God's Spirit rather than solely relying upon a written code.

For believers, *Shav'uot* signifies a "harvest" not of grain but of souls, symbolizing the abundant spiritual fruit that the Holy Spirit produces within and through the faithful. We celebrate *Shav'uot* as a profound expression of continuity and renewal that acknowledges both the foundational gift of the *Torah* and the transformational gift of the Holy Spirit, which together guide us into a life set apart for God.

Rosh Hashanah ["Head of the Year"] At A Glance

Traditional Celebration: *Rosh Hashanah*, alternatively known as the Feast of Trumpets is also the Jewish New Year and is celebrated with the blowing of the *shofar* ["ram's horn"] to mark the beginning of the Ten Days of Repentance. It is a day of introspection and judgment, as God is said to open the Book of Life to record the fates of His people.

Historical Significance: *Rosh Hashanah* is not only the Jewish New Year but also commemorates the creation of the world and emphasizes both God's rulership and His role as the ultimate Judge.

Spiritual Significance: The blowing of the *shofar* calls the community to repentance and reflection as it symbolizes a "wake-up call" for the soul. It is a time for the faithful to consider their relationship with God and others, and to make amends where necessary as it transitions into the solemn period of *Yom Kippur*.

Messianic Meaning: For the Messianic community, *Rosh Hashanah* holds additional eschatological significance. The blowing of the *shofar* is associated with Yeshua's triumphant return, as the trumpet will sound at His coming (1 Thessalonians 4:16).

The themes of repentance and judgment also reflect our hope in the Messiah's return and the ultimate fulfillment of God's kingdom on earth. (Isaiah 65:17; Revelation 21:1-4).

A Deeper Look At Rosh Hashanah ["Head of the Year"]

Rosh Hashanah, the Jewish New Year, marks the beginning of a sacred journey. It ushers us into the High Holy Days—a time of deep reflection, renewal, and repentance.

This holiday is an incredible blend of rejoicing and serious introspection, celebrating the gift of another year while beckoning us to examine our lives under the light of God's holiness.

According to Jewish tradition, the holiday commemorates creation, specifically the sixth day...the birthday of humanity. It is here, at the threshold of a new year, that we're invited to realign our hearts with God, to seek His direction, and to enter this season with a spirit of expectancy.

The two days of *Rosh Hashanah* open the *Aseret Yemei Teshuvah* [Ten Days of Repentance], also known as the *Yamim Noraim* [Days of Awe] that lead toward the climactic observance of *Yom Kippur* [Day of Atonement]. These are not merely days on a calendar; they are a divine call to examine our hearts.

For a month leading up to *Rosh Hashanah*, the *shofar* [ram horn] is blown, an ancient trumpet blast symbolically awakening us from spiritual slumber. It's a sacred summons to prepare our hearts for what's to come, culminating with the *Selichot* [special petitionary prayer], leading us into a season of renewed connection with God.

During *Rosh Hashanah*, Jew's believe that God opens the Books of Life and Death, judging humanity and then sealing everyone's fate on *Yom Kippur*. These days are believed to be an opportunity to repent, to confront our shortcomings, and to stand honestly before God.

The origin of *Rosh Hashanah* as a time of divine judgment and renewal is rooted in the royal enthronement rituals of ancient Israel. While Scripture doesn't explicitly describe *Rosh Hashanah* as either a "New Year" or "Day of Judgment," rabbinic tradition has imbued it with deep significance as the anniversary of creation—a reminder that God is both Creator and Judge.

Rosh Hashanah is celebrated on the first day of *Tishrei*, the seventh month of the Hebrew calendar. For this reason, Jews view it as the "Sabbath of the Year", a time of spiritual rest and restoration. Although this event occurred during the Babylonian Captivity, rabbinical scholars marked *Rosh Hashanah* as a day to commemorate God's creative and redemptive power.

It's a time to remember the holiness of our calling, and candles are lit to symbolize God's light bringing order to chaos, echoing Genesis 1:3 CJB, "Then God said, 'Let there be light'; and there was light."

The blessings and prayers of this holiday season, from the *Kiddush* ["holiness"] spoken over the wine to the *Shehecheyanu* [a prayer to celebrate special occasions], declare our gratitude for life, God's faithfulness, and the gift of new beginnings.

One of the cherished customs of *Rosh Hashanah* is dipping apples in honey, symbolizing the hope for a "sweet" new year. In these simple practices, the Jews found comfort and strength, trusting in God's goodness as they prayed, "May it be Your will, Eternal our God, that this be a good and sweet year for us."

Rosh Hashanah's customs and prayers unite us in reflection and hope, allowing us to release the burdens of the past year and embrace God's promises for the year to come.

For followers of Yeshua, *Rosh Hashanah* takes on even greater meaning as it reminds us of God's appointed times [Heb. *moadim*] described in Leviticus 23...*and how Yeshua fulfills each one*. The fall feasts, beginning with *Rosh Hashanah*, prefigure the ultimate redemption in Messiah's return illustrated in 1 Corinthians 15:52 CJB, "It will take but a moment, the blink of an eye, at the final shofar. For the shofar will sound, and the dead will be raised to live forever, and we too will be changed."

Celebrating Rosh Hashanah as followers of Yeshua isn't a departure from our faith; it's a deepening of it. In observing these holy days, we enter God's divine story, a journey of redemption that leads us closer to Him. *Rosh Hashanah* and the other feasts invite us to reflect, celebrate, and anticipate...helping us align our lives with God's rhythm.

And...with the full assurance that our names are written in Book of Life (Revelation 3:5)...we approach this season in gratitude, not fear, knowing that through Yeshua, we find safe refuge in God's unshakeable promises.

Yom Kippur [Day of Atonement] At A Glance

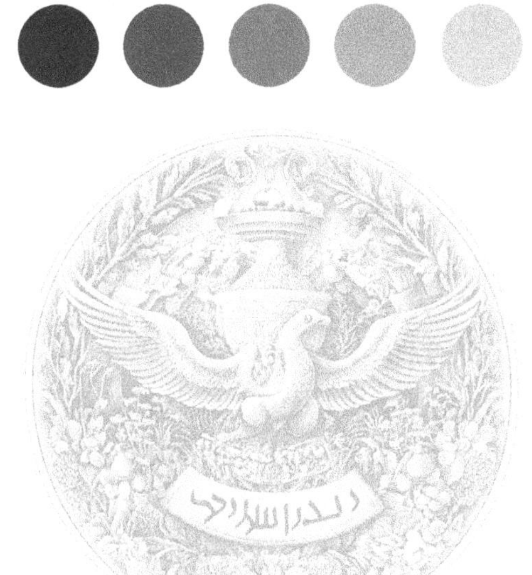

Traditional Celebration: *Yom Kippur* is observed as a solemn day of fasting and prayer and represents the culmination of the Ten Days of Repentance (which begin with *Rosh Hashanah*).

Traditionally, it was a day to seek forgiveness from both God and others for sins committed over the past year. Then, the high priest performed an elaborate ritual in the Temple to atone for the sins of Israel which included two goats. One would be sacrificed and the other (scapegoat) would be sent into the wilderness to symbolically bear the sins of Israel.

Historical Significance: *Yom Kippur* was instituted in Leviticus 16 and designated as the one day of the year when the high priest would be permitted to enter the Holy of Holies to atone for the sins of Israel. These sacrifices symbolized God's mercy in covering over sin and the renewal of His covenant relationship with Israel.

Spiritual Significance: *Yom Kippur* is the holiest day of the Jewish year and illustrates God's mercy and His willingness to forgive the repentant. It emphasizes the need for self-examination, repentance, and reconciliation with God. The celebration of *Yom Kippur* underscores one of the central themes in Scripture...that atonement is necessary for maintaining a relationship with God.

Messianic Meaning: For the Messianic community, *Yom Kippur* has been fulfilled through Yeshua whose death on the cross was the ultimate atonement for sin and represented the completion of the *Torah's* sacrificial system.

We now reflect on Yeshua as our High Priest (Hebrews 4:14-16) who entered the heavenly Holy of Holies (Hebrews 9) and fully atoned for the sins of humanity once and for all.

A Deeper Look At Yom Kippur [Day of Atonement]

In Leviticus 16, God describes the ritual to be performed by the *Cohen Gadol* [High Priest] to commemorate *Yom Kippur*.

The High Priest was instructed to offer a bull as his personal sin offering. He confessed his sins, those of his family, the sins of the tribe of Aaron [*Cohanim*], and then finally those of all Israel.

Every time the High Priest uttered the holy name of God [the *Tetragrammaton*], which was only spoken on *Yom Kippur*, the people prostrated themselves and responded: “Praised is His name, whose glorious kingdom is forever and ever.”

Lots were drawn to determine which of the two male goats would be sent into the wilderness for Azazel, and which one would be sacrificed as a sin offering for the Lord. After a special incense offering was made in the Holy of Holies, the High Priest recited a prayer blessing Israel with peace, prosperity, and fertility.

Yom Kippur is the heart of the year, the holiest day in God’s calendar—a sacred pause when heaven meets earth in a profound way. Traditionally, on this Day of Atonement, the high priest entered the Holy of Holies to seek forgiveness for Israel’s sins.

We experience this day as an invitation to remember that Yeshua, our eternal High Priest, offered the ultimate sacrifice on our behalf. His blood covers every sin, every wound, every moment of failure...and releases us from striving to “earn” forgiveness while calling us to receive what he has already freely and fully given to us.

The invitation of *Yom Kippur* goes much deeper than just tradition; it’s a call to introspection, a journey into the shadows of our hearts. It isn’t about punishment or self-condemnation but about “tearing the curtain” to see ourselves honestly and confront our tendency to rationalize our beliefs and justify our actions...to think we are “right”, even when we are not.

It is part of our human nature to engage in self-deception from time to time as we cling to a version of ourselves that does not align with God's truth. On *Yom Kippur*, God opens the door to that deeper awareness and offers us a choice...walk through to discover who we are and who He made us to be...or look away.

For some, *Yom Kippur* includes fasting as a way to deliberately step away from the usual distractions of life and to realign with God's heart. Fasting is a sacred reminder that *our deepest need is for His presence*...not mere physical sustenance. It represents our desire to be filled, not just with food, but with the fullness of His love. Fasting reminds us that, through Yeshua, we have access to the Holy of Holies—*the very presence of God*. A place where guilt and shame give way to grace, and we are free to walk in the light of His love.

The essence of *Yom Kippur* is reconciliation—between God, ourselves, and others. It calls for releasing ourselves and others from the chains of resentment...mirroring the grace we've received through Yeshua. This is the power of "at-one-ment"...the healing of the separation caused by sin.

The Hebrew word *korban* ["sacrifice"] means "to draw near" which perfectly describes Yeshua's sacrifice that draws us close, bridges the chasm, and invites us to be co-heirs to God's promises (Romans 8:17).

Yom Kippur is also about *teshuvah,* a continual and lifelong process of turning away from sin and returning to God in order to reclaim our truest identity in Him. As we extend forgiveness, it creates more space for His peace to fill our hearts. *Yom Kippur* invites us to a life marked by reconciliation and renewal. Through Yeshua's atonement we are empowered by the Holy Spirit to experience his gift of grace and step forward into his story for our lives.

Sukkot [Feast of Tabernacles] At A Glance

Traditional Celebration: *Sukkot*, also known as the Feast of Tabernacles or Booths, is a seven-day celebration that begins on the 15th day of *Tishrei*. Traditionally, Jewish families built a *sukkah* ["booths" or "hut"] and lived in it for the duration. The *sukkah* served as a reminder of the temporary dwellings of the Israelites during their 40 years of wandering in the wilderness.

During the celebration, special prayers and blessings are recited, including the waving of the *lulav* ["palm branch"], *etrog* ["citron"], *hadass* ["myrtle"], and *aravah* ["willow"], known as the Four Species. These symbolize different parts of creation and the unity of God's people. *Sukkot* also features festive meals, hospitality, and communal worship in the synagogue.

Historical Significance: *Sukkot* commemorates the Israelites' time in the wilderness following their exodus from Egypt and reminds them of God's protection and provision during those forty years when they lived in temporary shelters. Moreover, *Sukkot* was also an agricultural festival that marked the end of the harvest season and offered gratitude for God's provision of food and shelter. This dual theme—God's provision both historically (in the wilderness) and agriculturally (through the harvest)—is a central theme of the celebration.

Spiritual Significance: *Sukkot* represents God's presence and provision for His people, and the temporary nature of the *sukkah* symbolizes human dependence on God and the fragile nature of life. True security and sustenance comes from God alone. The feast also reflects a time of joy as the Israelites were instructed to rejoice before the LORD (Leviticus 23:40).

Messianic Meaning: For the Messianic community, *Sukkot* foreshadows the Messianic Kingdom, where God's presence will dwell among His people in a

even more completely when someday, all nations will celebrate the Feast of Tabernacles (Zechariah 14:16) together. We also reflect how Yeshua was "The Word became a human being and lived with us," (John 1:14).

In this context, the phrase, "lived with us" (Strong's G4637) means "tabernacle" and signifies that the physical incarnation of Yeshua is God's ultimate dwelling among His people. Additionally, *Sukkot* points to the Messiah's future reign, when all of humanity will live under God's protection and we will celebrate the final harvest at the end of time.

A Deeper Look At Sukkot [Feast of Tabernacles]

Beginning five days after *Yom Kippur*, *Sukkot* ["tent" or "booth"] marks the beginning of a week-long celebration in which Jews are supposed to dwell in tents. According to rabbinic tradition, the flimsy *sukkot* represents the tents in which the Israelites dwelt during their forty years of wandering in the desert after escaping from slavery in Egypt.

The feast of *Sukkot* originated in the celebration of an ancient autumnal harvest festival. This is why it is often referred to as *hag ha-asif* ["The Harvest Festival."] For that reason, much of the imagery and ritual of the holiday revolves around rejoicing and thanking God for the completed harvest.

The *sukkah* represented the temporary tents or huts that farmers lived in during the final harvest period before the winter rains. Thus, *Sukkot* commemorates the forty years of wandering in the desert that the Israelites experienced following God's revelation at Mount Sinai, with the huts representing the temporary shelters they lived in during that time.

Many of the most popular rituals of *Sukkot* are practiced in the home. As close to the conclusion of *Yom Kippur* as possible (often that same evening), one begins building a *sukkah*. As the central symbol of the festival, this flimsy structure has at least three sides with a roof made from thatch or branches.

The object of the structure is to provide protection from the sun while still being able to see the stars at night.

According to tradition, as the *sukkah* is decorated, during the intermediate days of *Sukkot*, one is allowed to pursue normal activity while spending as much time as possible in the structure. Weather permitting, meals are eaten in the *sukkah*, and some even choose to sleep in it.

The simplicity of eating and possibly living in a temporary shelter shifts one's focus to the essentials of life, freeing the heart and mind from the dominance of modern material possessions.

Even so, *Sukkot* is a joyful holiday and described as *zeman simchateynu* ["season of our joy"].

The Scriptures clearly record Yeshua and his followers celebrating the festivals, including *Sukkot*. Everything he did and said was completely aligned with Scripture and offers us a glimpse into his union with the Father. Moreover, understanding where and when his words were spoken, allow for a new depth of meaning and significance.

Imagine being at the Feast of *Sukkot*: the temporary dwellings, fragrant smells of the harvest, the waving of the four species, and a celebration full of joyful gratitude. Now...picture Yeshua standing among the people and speaking these words recorded in the book of John:

> **JOHN 7:7 CJB** | 7 The world can't hate you, but it does hate me [Yeshua], because I keep telling it how wicked its ways are.

Observing the biblical feasts like *Sukkot* can feel awkward and out of place in today's world. But while stores decorate for Halloween and neighbors might raise an eyebrow at your *sukkah*...this week takes full aim at the cultural norms of both society and the modern Church.

Yeshua lived his entire life as a witness against the world system...and when we choose his ways, we too become that witness.

> **JOHN 7:8 CJB** | 8 You, go on up to the festival [Sukkot]; as for me, I [Yeshua] am not going up to this festival now, because the right time for me has not yet come."

Notice that Yeshua didn't add, "...if it's convenient" to verse 8 as he urged his brothers to celebrate the Feast of Tabernacles. Also, keep in mind that *Sukkot* is a *seven-day* festival requiring time, resources, and a 70-mile journey from Galilee to Jerusalem.

> **JOHN 7:16 CJB** | [16] So Yeshua [Jesus] gave them [the Judeans] an answer: "My teaching is not my own, it comes from the One who sent me."

Yeshua's reminder that his teachings align with God's commands also meant that what God desired...he desired. Since God established *Sukkot*, Yeshua gladly and joyously obeyed his Father's command to celebrate the festival.

> **JOHN 7:23 CJB** | [23] "If a boy is circumcised on Shabbat [Sabbath] so that the Torah [Law] of Moshe [Moses] will not be broken, why are you angry with me because I made a man's whole body well on Shabbat?

After his miraculous act of healing on the Sabbath during *Sukkot*, Yeshua was accused of being under demonic possession. Though some of the Judeans misunderstood this as violation of *Torah*, it wasn't *Torah* that Yeshua violated...but rather, their *man-made rules*. Similarly, when we strive to live our lives for God, we may face criticism (or worse), but Yeshua calls us to remain faithful to Scripture without bending to the expectations of the world.

> **JOHN 7:24 CJB** | [24] Stop judging by surface appearances and judge the right way!"

Although this verse is often abbreviated to "Do not judge", Yeshua's full teaching encourages us to *discern rightly*. We are called to evaluate actions *according to Scripture*, not outward appearances. When understood correctly, righteous judgment is a necessary tool for interpreting both Scripture and our own lives.

> **JOHN 7:37 CJB** | [37] Now on the last day of the festival, Hoshana Rabbah [seventh day of Sukkot], Yeshua [Jesus] stood and cried out, "If anyone is thirsty, let him keep coming to me and drinking!"

Yeshua's beautiful invitation to refresh and revive those who come to him is even more meaningful when we realize that if you wanted to go to Him, you would have had to be celebrating at the Feast of *Sukkot*.

> **JOHN 7:38 CJB** | [38] "Whoever puts his trust in me [Yeshua], as the Scripture says, rivers of living water will flow from his inmost being!"

Yeshua was stating that the Scriptures (Genesis through Malachi) all point to him and that even the feasts are part of this divine testimony. So, why would we overlook anything that reveals more of Yeshua's heart?

Ultimately, we are invited to follow his example into deep intimacy and union with God.

As a quick reminder, Scripture reveals that during *Sukkot*, Yeshua:

- Went to the Temple in Jerusalem for the festival (John 7:2).
- Encouraged others to attend the festival (John 7:8).
- Attended the festival himself (John 7:10).
- Taught the people (John 7:14).

> **1 JOHN 2:3-6 CJB** | [3] The way we can be sure we know him is if we are obeying his commands. [4] Anyone who says, "I know him," but isn't obeying his commands is a liar — the truth is not in him. [5] But if someone keeps doing what he says, then truly love for God has been brought to its goal in him. This is how we are sure that we are united with him. [6] A person who claims to be continuing in union with him ought to conduct his life the way he did.

If we choose to take our relationship with Yeshua seriously, then we are called to walk as he did—honoring the heart (not the Law) of the feasts, keeping God's commands, and loving Him with all of our heart, mind, soul, and strength.

Sukkot, like the other appointed times is not just a Hebrew tradition...it's a reflection of our Messiah's life and his love for God's ways.

THRIVE ON

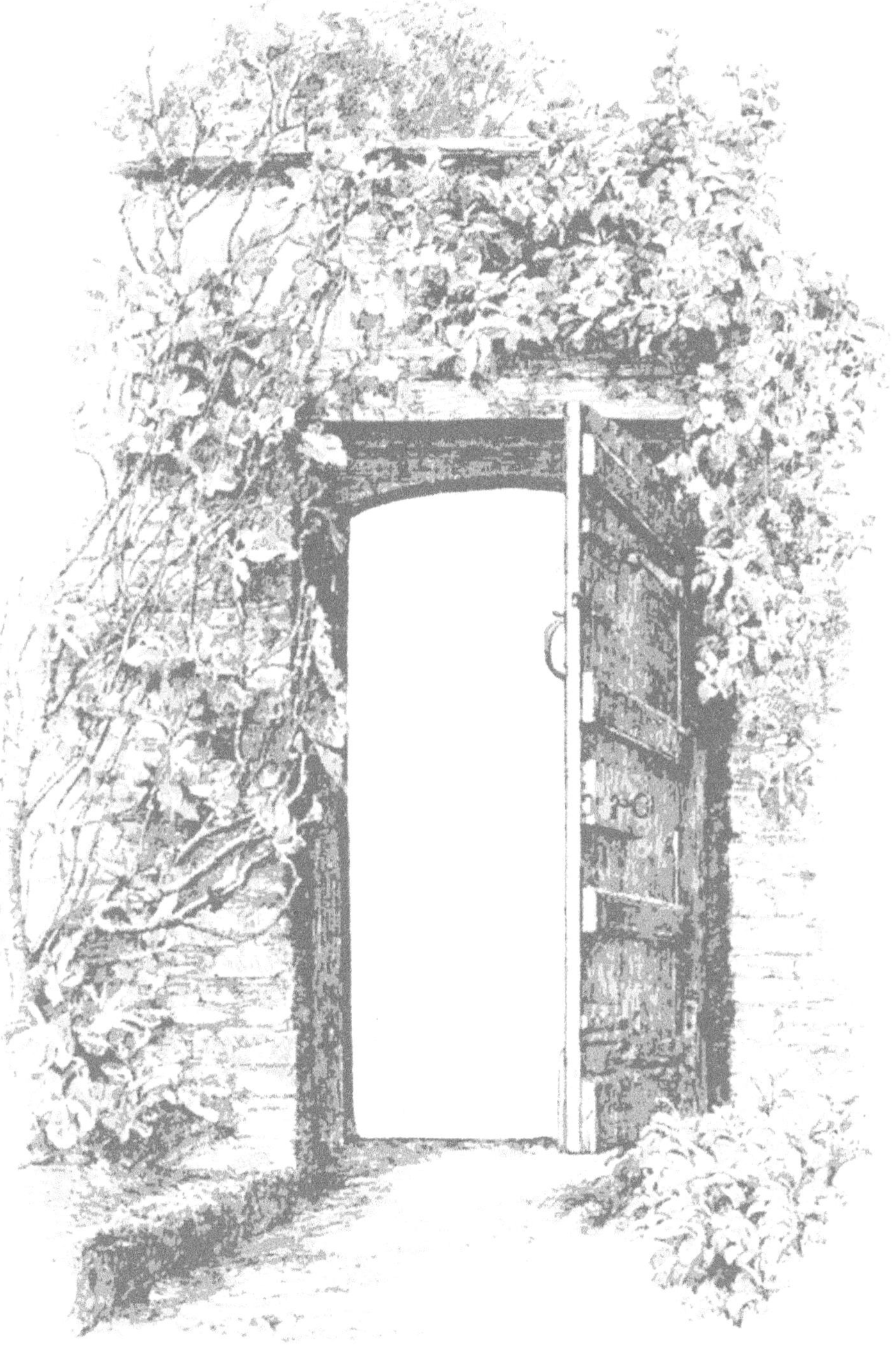

Part 6

THRIVE ON

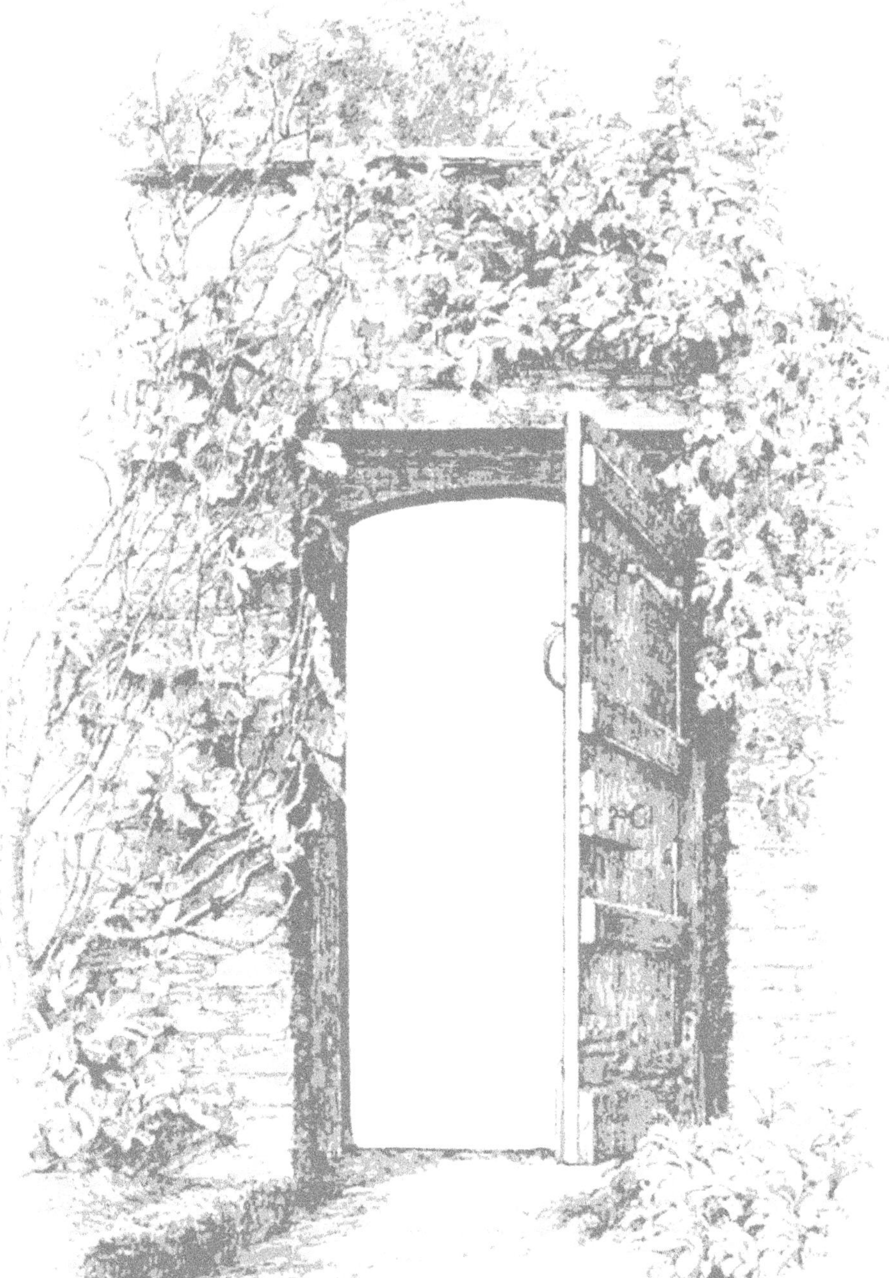

Part 6

The Scriptures are very clear that each month of the year is endowed with prophetic significance. That is why God arranged the weeks, months, and years into seasons...so that as we walk with Him, week by week, month by month, year by year...we're able to *remain aligned to His purposes for our lives.*

Part of walking in God's presence is centering our lives around His calendar and embracing the rhythms He has established for our time.

The more aligned we are with God, the more we fully live in sync with His timing...and will make the most of His windows of opportunity.

At the end of every season, *we must intentionally shift from our current position to our destined position*...and we hope that you are moving there even as you read these words. ☺

As the scale of this guide continues to grow, we will be adding monthly teachings on the Sabbath, Hebrew months, and High Holy Days. Our desire is to explore how, as followers of Yeshua, we can grow closer to God and increasingly experience His presence!

Inspired Life Membership Manifesto

The Inspired Life Movement was created as a sanctuary for spiritual growth, personal transformation, emotional wellness, and relational support in community with Spirit-driven, like-minded people. If you are wondering if our group would be a good fit for you, this is who we are...

Inspired Lifers are committed to pursuing an intimate union with God and to bring Him into every aspect of their lives. To that end, they seek alignment with God's daily rhythms and seasons to experience the fullness of His purpose.

Inspired Lifers don't dwell on obstacles; instead, they view them as God's training program for the possibilities that lie ahead and are willing to faithfully follow wherever the Holy Spirit leads.

Inspired Lifers dream, plan, and live according to God's design.

They are life-long learners dedicated to spiritual, emotional, and mental growth. They embrace the reality that maturity and whole-heartedness are not optional.

Inspired Lifers understand that our journey with God is infinite, and that a deeper understanding of Him is a forever process that allows for better questions that foster greater connection and clarity.

Inspired Lifers are eager to help others and deliver more value than expected.

Inspired Lifers champion their own dreams as well as the dreams of others. They vulnerably share their authentic selves and reject the facade of living a false life.

Inspired Lifers are fully invested in God's incredible inheritance and calling. They inspire others with their passion and choose to live in His truth and freedom.

If this resonates in your spirit, we would love for you to join us.

Here are some of the ways you can stay connected and continue your momentum!

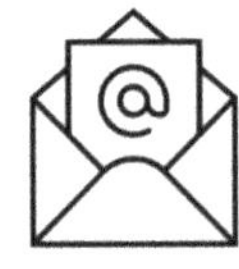

Join our email list (if you haven't already) to receive regular (but not spammy) updates on all the latest.

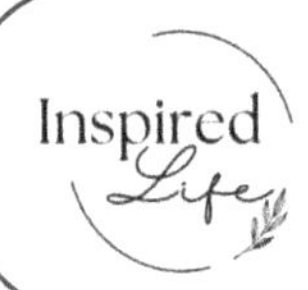

Become an Inspired Lifer and join a thriving Messianic community of like-minded believers who are committed to seeking alignment and deeper union with God. www.inspiredlifemovement.com/membership

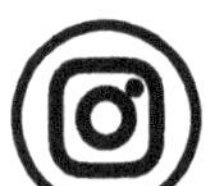 @freedomfromgrief

 @danielhagadorn

 calendly.com/freedomfromgrief
Vicki

 calendly.com/one-on-one-consultation/30-min
Daniel

We curated this list from the best resources we've found—tools that God has used bring deeper growth, encouragement, inspiration and learning into our lives.

עידוד　למידה　השראה

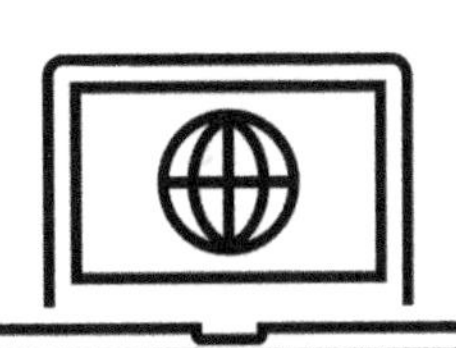

- **Curt Landry Ministries** @ curtlandry.com
- **Fusion with Rabbi Jason** @ fusionglobal.org
- **The Bible Project** @ bibleproject.com
- **Troy Brewer** @ troybrewer.com
- **John Eldredge** @ wildatheart.org
- **Chuck Pierce** @ kingofkingswc.com

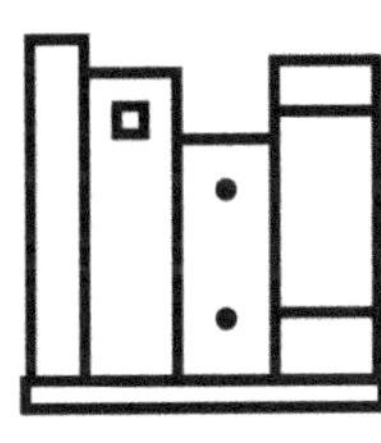

- **The Sacred Romance** by Brent Curtis & John Eldredge
- **Walking With God** by John Eldredge
- **The Unseen Realm** by Michael S. Heiser
- **A Family Guide To Biblical Holidays** by Robin Scarletta & Linda Pierce
- **Emotionally Healthy Spirituality** by Peter Scazzero

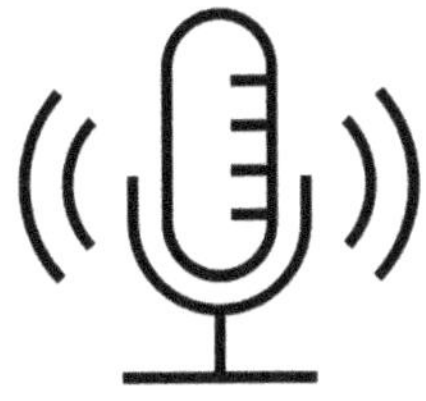

- **Wild At Heart Podcast** @ wildatheart.org
- **The BEMA Podcast** @ bemadiscipleship.com
- **The Naked Bible Podcast** @ nakedbiblepodcast.com
- **360 Parenting Blog & Podcast** @ pk4l.substack.com

Shalom!

www.ingramcontent.com/pod-product-compliance
Lightning Source LLC
Chambersburg PA
CBHW080643270326
41928CB00017B/3176
9780999282779